Ashtanga Yoga

for all those who practise
&
for all those who are yet to practise

Ashtanga Yoga

Richard Pilnick

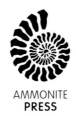

AMMONITE
PRESS

Contents

The Asanas
6

A Gift of Photography
8

A Guide to the Book
11

Origins and Practices
12

THE PRACTICE

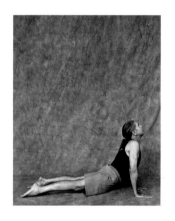

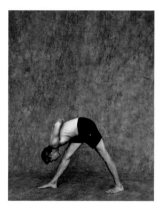

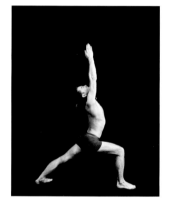

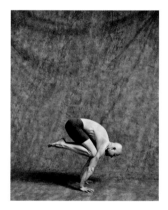

Sun Salutation A & B
David Williams
16

Fundamental Positions
Gingi Lee
36

Primary
John Scott
50

Intermediate
Ronald Steiner
96

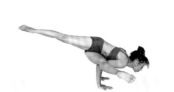

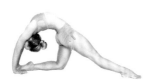

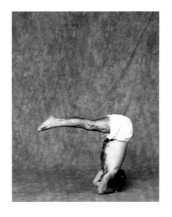

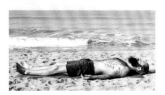

Advanced A
Laruga Glaser
138

Advanced B
Kino MacGregor
186

Finishing Sequence
Danny Paradise
252

Shavasana
Richard Pilnick
272

The Teachers
278

Acknowledgments
288

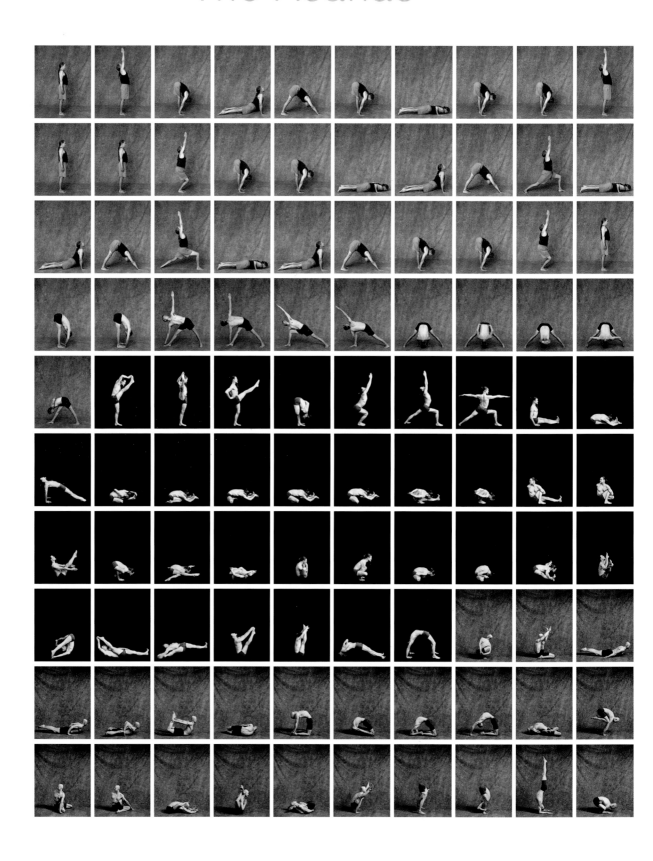

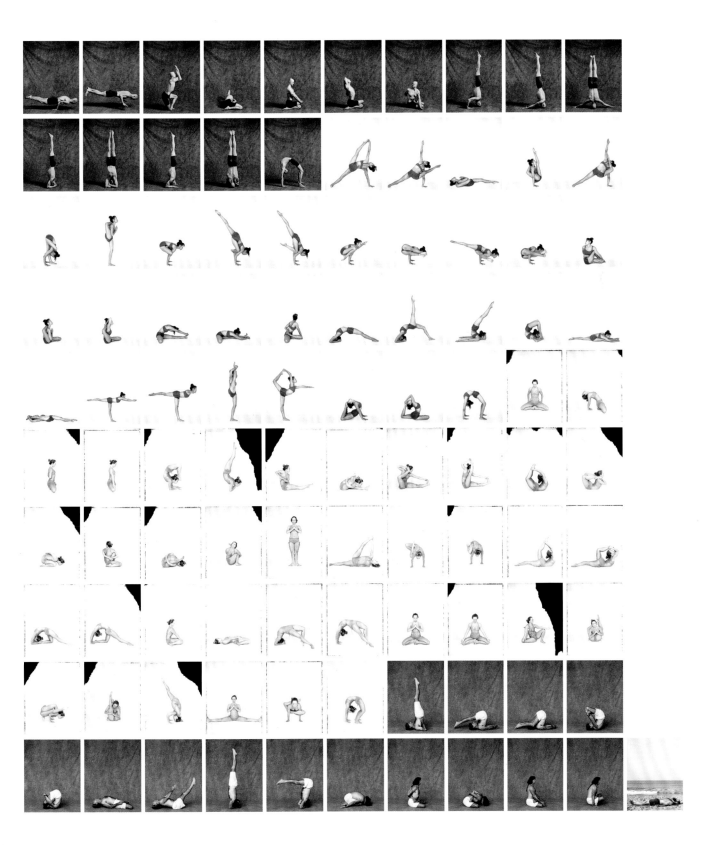

7

A Gift of Photography

Ashtanga changed my life. In 2008, I was working within the fashion industry, fulfilling all my ambitions and yet feeling far from fulfilled. I decided I needed to take some time out, to get some perspective and ensure that I was creating images from my heart and not just shooting what I thought people wanted to see. So, I packed my bags and headed to India for two months. In Jodhpur, the blue city, I had my first yoga session on a rooftop: half an hour of Sun Salutations to the rising sun, followed by a ginger black tea while philosophizing about life and flying kites with the local kids. At the time I was reading Khaled Hosseini's *The Kite Runner*, so it felt almost like I was in Kabul.

We headed south to Karnataka, to the small village of Gokarna, for three days, which quickly turned into a month. Captivated by the people, both local and foreign, I decided I wanted to capture the essence of this beautiful space through their eyes. I went into the village and managed to get all the supplies I needed to build a pop-up studio on the beach: some 12-foot bamboo poles from the guest house where we were staying; rope and a sickle from the hardware store; and a local hammock-maker shaped me a 20 x 20-foot white sheet for diffusing the sunlight and a black sheet for negative fill. I also found some rice sacks, which I filled with sand to weigh everything down.

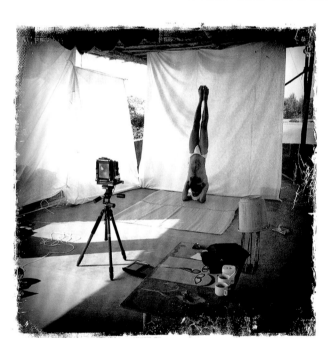

Beach studio, Gokarna, 2011

The next day, on 2 January 2009 at 5.30 a.m., my alarm sounded. It wasn't actually needed as I hadn't slept due to my feeling of excitement. I dragged all the materials down to the beach and began building the studio. An hour later, as I struggled on the beach, a group of men came over and started helping me to finalize the structure, even though they had no idea what I was doing or why. But when it was all finished and I got my camera out, they were all fighting to be first for a picture and were exchanging clothes with each other to ensure that they looked their best. At that time, I was shooting on a Hasselblad 500, a medium-format camera. So popular was the studio, that I shot around 35 rolls of film on that first day. Someone even swam the length of the beach to see what was going on.

But there was one face and one photograph that changed everything for me. It has since been studied by Eric Standop, a face reader from Germany, who wrote a poem that gave the image its name, and I now refer to the subject of the portrait as 'Sad Eyes'. Unable to communicate, and with no knowledge of who I was or what I was doing, he had waited patiently with his bags to present himself to me for a portrait. We shared only a brief moment together, which transcended verbal communication. When I returned to London, this was the first picture that struck me. Captivated by this image (it was the first print I had made) I had a moment of clarity and of realization – I was a portrait photographer, and this was the journey I needed to take.

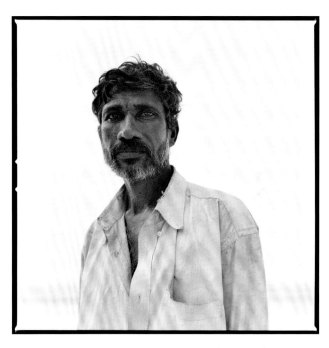

'Sad Eyes', Gokarna, 2009

I quit everything. I spoke to all my clients and all the other photographers I was working for at the time and told them I was leaving. I ended up spending three and a half years living and working in Asia, returning to Gokarna on numerous occasions. Every time I visit the village, I take prints from the previous portrait session, and I am always in search of 'Sad Eyes'. It's a small village where everyone knows everyone, yet nobody knows who he is or where he is from. He is my guardian angel, he presented himself to me for me to realize my destiny and purpose. Every day I ask myself, was he really there?

In 2012, in Malaysia, I sat down with Eric to reflect upon my life up until that point: the work I had done, the pictures I had taken and the inspiration that had led me to take a series of photographs of the Indian yogi, Shiva Shankar, in the same village of Gokarna. It had all been built upon the same foundation: yoga. If that was going to be the direction I wanted to take, then I needed to photograph more yoga.

Returning to London I introduced myself to Cat Alip-Douglas, an experienced yoga teacher and co-director of Sangyé Yoga, formerly Jivamukti Yoga London, and asked if we could shoot together. Inspired by my portraiture, she happily accepted. I took two frames of Cat with her husband, Phil, but I knew immediately that they were wrong. They didn't feel connected with the situation and the camera.

So we changed things around, and I took one more photograph. That picture ended up not only being exhibited in London's National Portrait Gallery, but also displayed as a huge poster on the outside of the building, showcasing

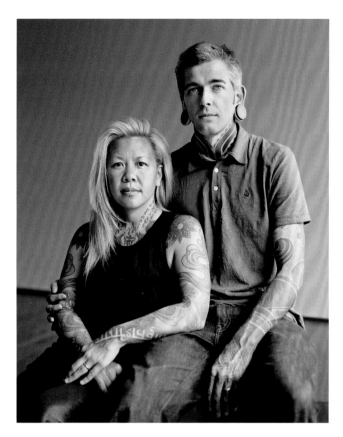

Cat and Phil Alip-Douglas, London, 2012

the Taylor Wessing Portrait Prize. I was on the right path; I had received a nod and a wink from the Universe.

It was not until the following year that I found Ashtanga yoga. I had tried various practices but it was back in the village of Gokarna, with teacher Marco Aicardi, that I found my connection. Concentrating on the breath, in the silence of the practice, calmed my mind. It made me more focused, more connected to myself, and it helped me to form a new relationship with my inner self, my soul.

Ashtanga helped me to find my inner self, so I wanted to pay homage to Ashtanga through my gift of photography. As a portrait photographer, people have always fascinated me. Faces of this world have driven me to travel throughout Asia and the Far East in search of beauty, in the true sense of the word – the beauty of the soul, shining inside and out. I spoke to John Scott about this project and his words helped to clarify my thoughts: 'See that beauty that you're seeing outside and see if you can see that on the inside... for me, that's where the yoga really starts to go from the one where your mind is being drawn outward, maybe distracted by all the stimulus out there; the *pratyahara* is to know that the beauty exists out there only because of what comes from the inside. So, then we are guided by our practice to look in…'

I am a fine-art portrait photographer who uses large-format cameras in a meditative and mindful way to try to capture that true beauty, that essence of being, the soul. So, yoga photography for me is about honouring the practice by bringing integrity back to the images used to portray the practice. It is also about inspiration – inspiring more people into the practice through the medium of photographic art.

Yoga has the ability to heal. Yoga has the ability to bring about peace. So, the more people we can inspire to practise, the happier and healthier this world will become.

Richard Pilnick

A Guide to the Book

This book is both an in-depth photographic celebration of Ashtanga (aṣṭāṅga) yoga and an authoritative sourcebook of the series, sequences, names and forms of the asanas. It is not intended as a step-by-step guide, but rather as a comprehensive and definitive visual reference for the essential elements of the practice.

The asanas

The book presents a course of study for the Ashtanga asanas or postures. Each chapter demonstrates a specific series of asanas in their prescribed sequence. First are the Sun Salutation A & B and Fundamental Postures. These are followed by the Primary and Intermediate series. Next come the higher levels of difficulty in the first two Advanced series, Advanced A & B, with Advanced B being showcased here for the first time. And the book concludes with the Finishing sequence. The final image shows the photographer in the Śavāsana, or Corpse Pose, where the practitioner is intended to be both fully conscious and completely relaxed as they assimilate the benefits of the completed practice – just as the reader is invited to look back on the book's images.

The teachers

Each series is demonstrated by a leading teacher from the international community, all of whom have used their work to inspire and develop generations of Ashtanga teachers and practitioners. In their chapter, each teacher demonstrates a definitive sequence of the asanas in the series. Biographies of the teachers can be found on pages 278–87.

The photography

The images were all photographed using a large-format film camera and black-and-white film to present the mindful and meditative beauty of Ashtanga yoga in a detail that literally catches the breath. The contrasting backdrops were selected for the different series to reflect the photographer's own personal journey through light and darkness. The Advanced B series was shot on old Polaroid film to create its unique texture and to allow the decay of the film to manifest itself in random combinations of light and shadow, postive and negative.

The Sanskrit and transliteration

The names of the asanas are transcribed in their Western and transliterated forms, as well as in the Sanskrit, to provide a complete reference source of terms to accompany the photography. All terminology has been provided by Ronald Steiner and written to accord with the online resources available at www.ashtangayoga.info.

The poems

Alongside the portrait photograph of the teacher demonstrating the asanas, each chapter begins with a personal poem written for the teacher by the face reader Eric Standop. Eric studies his subjects to offer insights into their characters, and to encourage self-understanding and acceptance, and he was the source of the name 'Sad Eyes' bestowed upon the original photograph that inspired Richard Pilnick's aṣṭāṅga yoga journey which resulted in the images that are at the heart of this book.

Origins and Practices

Various dates have been proposed for the origin of yoga. The truth is that no one really knows; yoga practices may be ten thousand years old or perhaps date from only around two and a half thousand years ago.

The earliest materials that might indicate yoga practices in South Asia are seals that come from the Indus Valley civilization (2300–1600 BCE), depicting what have been called 'proto-Śiva' images (Śiva being one of the great gods of Hinduism). These seals, which were made of steatite or soapstone, were attached to packages being traded or transported and were imprinted with various images of animals and trees and a script, which to this day remains undeciphered. The 'proto-Śiva' images are of someone seated in what may or may not be a yoga posture; scholars are divided over whether or not they indicate the practice of postural yoga.

The notion of brahman

In the cultures of South Asia and Greece, as in nearly all other human cultures, there were mythological accounts of the origins of the world and of the deeds of deities, but it was not until around 700 BCE that philosophy first properly developed in both India and Greece. By 'philosophy', what is meant here is primarily the enquiry into the difference between appearance and reality. This requires the capacity for abstract thinking – about things that one cannot actually see – an aspect of which is being able to conceive of an invisible power: whether that be the 'God' of the Judeo-Christian world, or the idea in South Asia of a cosmic power known as 'brahman' underlying reality, which began to crystallize around this time.

This notion of brahman first properly appears in the Upaniṣads, which are semi-philosophical, partly poetical texts that date from around 700 BCE and form the final section of the Vedas. The Vedas are the oldest of the sacred texts of Hinduism, dating back to around 1600 BCE, in which the most important sections contain mantras that are recited for religious rituals.

In the Upaniṣads, embedded typically in conversations between priests and kings, there are some passages of discussions on the nature of brahman. Questions are posed about the relationship between oneself (ātman) and brahman, what happens after death, what happens to the five airs or winds in the body after death, and the nature of the Self. In four of the twelve (or thirteen) of the classical Upaniṣads (the Taittirīya, Kaṭha, Maitrī and Svetâsvatara Upaniṣads) there are also passages that for the first time in the tradition discuss yoga as a spiritual practice. They speak of the mind and senses needing to be controlled to attain liberation from engagement with the external world and repeated rounds of rebirth. Of prime importance are meditation and either the control or observation of the breath, practices that are the foundations of yoga.

Between around 600 and 400 BCE there arose in South Asia two new religions that flourished and are still practised widely today, Jainism and Buddhism. Similarly to the practices of yoga referred to in the Upaniṣads, of central importance in Buddhism and

Jainism are yogic practices of meditation, providing insights into the true nature of reality and liberation from our habitual engagement with the world.

Aṣṭāṅga – the yoga of eight limbs

Today, the best-known text on yoga is the Yoga Sūtra of Patañjali, which was composed between around 375 CE and 425 CE. It was written in Sanskrit and has been translated more often than any other Sanskrit text. A considerable Buddhist influence on the text may be discerned; there are concepts and terms borrowed directly from Buddhism, some in Buddhist Sanskrit. The sūtras are traditionally read or recited alongside the earliest of the commentaries on the Yoga Sūtra, the commentary (bhāṣya) by Vyāsa. However, 'Vyāsa' means 'editor' or 'compiler' and we don't really know who Vyāsa was. The combined sūtras and the commentary by Vyāsa are known as the Patañjalayogaśāstra. Recent work on this text by scholars indicates that both the sūtras and the earliest commentary by Vyāsa were written by Patañjali himself, though not all scholars agree with this idea.

The system of the Yoga Sūtra is known as aṣṭāṅga yoga, the 'yoga of eight limbs / subsidiaries'. Patañjali defines yoga, in the second sūtra of his text, as the stopping of the movement (or turning) of the mind. In order to achieve this, he outlines an eight-fold, step-by-step path.

Firstly, the practising yogi must adhere to basic rules of ethics, in the form of restraints (yamas) and observances (niyamas). These are the first two limbs, comprising non-violence, truth, not stealing, remaining celibate, and not being greedy (the five yamas); and cleanliness, contentment, performing austerities, recitation of the Vedas on one's own, and concentrating on the Lord (the five niyamas).

The yogi is then in a sufficiently harmonious state of mind to be able to sit steadily and comfortably. This is āsana, the third limb. Vyāsa lists a dozen different positions that the meditator may comfortably adopt. (It was only around 1000 CE that the term āsana began to be used as a term referring to more strenuous standing postures.)

The yogi then begins breath control (prāṇāyāma), the fourth limb, which leads gradually to a concentration on the breath and the withdrawal of the senses from the external world. This is known as pratyāhāra, the fifth limb.

There then arise progressively deeper states of meditation, the first being dhāraṇā, the sixth limb, in which an object such as a candle is concentrated upon. The next stage is meditation practised without an object, which is dhyāna, the seventh limb. The eighth limb is the deepest state of meditation, samādhi, which is perhaps best described as a state of trance, in which the yogi undergoes a near-death experience. This state has similarities with the state of hibernation, which some animals can enter into.

Samādhi is an ecstatic, blissful experience in which the negative impressions that have been accumulated and colour the mind are eradicated. It is also referred to as a state of 'aloneness' (kaivalya), in which the only thing of which the meditator is aware is pure consciousness (puruṣa); the mind, body and senses, and the external world (all of which are prakṛti), fade from awareness.

Heightened states

According to Patañjali, a by-product of the practice of yoga is the acquisition of occult powers, which are known as siddhis or vibhūtis. Patañjali lists around twenty-five powers that may arise as a result of concentration on various parts of the body (such as the navel cakra or the throat); on features of the cosmos (such as the sun or the moon); or on the senses. These powers are specified in the third chapter (the Vibhūti Pāda) of the Yoga Sūtra and include clairvoyance, knowing the time of one's death, and the powers to become invisible, enter another's body, levitate, or become very large or very small.

One way of understanding these kinds of powers is to consider them as extensions of our natural capacities, rather than as 'magical' or impossible. Non-ordinary states of consciousness are frequently associated with a heightened sense of premonition or telepathy. It does need to be emphasized that in the traditional world of yoga in India, yoga was generally practised not only to attain liberation but also to acquire such 'powers'.

Tantra and Hatha yoga

From around the 6th century CE, systems of ritual and meditation practice known broadly as Tantra or Tantric yoga, which had both Hindu and Buddhist expressions, developed in South Asia and spread gradually throughout Asia. One of the metaphysical innovations in Tantra was the elaboration of the well-known 'Tantric body', comprising variously a scheme of either four, five, six, seven or nine (or more) cakras (wheels) located in the body; nāḍīs (psychic channels conducting energy within the body); and kuṇḍalinī, the coiled serpent of female energy (śakti) which, when aroused, rises up from the base of the spine, piercing the cakras, to unite eventually with the pure (male) consciousness, mostly personified as Śiva, at a point just above the crown of the head.

From around the 11th or 12th centuries, these Tantric notions fused with the older practices of yoga, namely meditation, celibacy and breath control. In the medieval period this fusion of practices and concepts was broadly conceived of as haṭha yoga, the yoga of 'force' or 'exertion'. Yoga texts of this period elaborate various methods to arouse kuṇḍalinī, including a range of practices to clean and purify the body and various routines of strenuous prāṇāyāma, and they describe many yoga postures (āsanas). It was only with the advent of Haṭha yoga that standing yoga postures were developed.

One of the best-known medieval texts on Haṭha yoga is the Haṭhapradīpikā (or Haṭhayogapradīpikā) by Svātmārāma, a text dating from the 15th century, which was compiled from more than a dozen earlier texts. Interestingly, it seems that it was Buddhist adepts who, around the 11th century, were among the pioneers of the practices of Haṭha yoga, which were developed with the primary aim of attaining powers and liberation while alive.

The modern lineages

In the 20th century, a significant turn in the development and spread of yoga practices occurred in Mysore, India. Between 1933 and 1950, the great yogi Krishnamacharya (1888–1989) taught at the yoga śālā in the Jaganmohan Palace in Mysore. Several of his students, including his son T.K.V. Desikachar (1938–2016), B.K.S. Iyengar (1918–2014), Indra Devi (1899–2002) and K. Pattabhi Jois (1915–2009), toured extensively abroad during their lifetimes, taking the practice of postural yoga worldwide. Krishnamacharya's lineage accounts for about half of the postural yoga practised in the world.

Besides this lineage, other schools that have been most influential in the spread of postural yoga are the Divine Life Society, based near Rishikesh, India, and founded by Swami Sivananda Saraswati (1887–1963); and the Bihar school of yoga, founded by Swami Satyananda Saraswati (1923–2009), who was formerly a student of Sivananda. Another influential lineage, originally from Calcutta, India, is that of Paramahansa Yogananda (1893–1952), who taught meditation but very little postural yoga, and Bikram Choudhury (b. 1944), who developed 'hot yoga'.

All of these teachers taught yoga practices differently, with varying degrees of emphasis on meditation, devotional chanting, bodily cleansing routines, prāṇāyāma, and postural practice. Pattabhi Jois developed a style of yoga practice he called aṣṭāṅga, adopting the name from Patañjali's system. Jois' system combines the ethics and meditation practice of Patañjali with a vigorous routine of postural exercises. The style is one of the more aerobic forms of yoga practice, involving the performance of a relatively large number of postures during a session. There are six series of postures (āsanas), arranged in three levels of practice, and they are performed in synchronization with even, rhythmic breathing. Also taught is a set of internal 'locks', known as bandhas; and, beginning with the practice of the second series of postures, various routines of prāṇāyāma.

These aṣṭāṅga yoga practices raise heat in the body, increase general strength and train the practitioner in the discipline of concentration on the breath and the internal control of particular muscle-groups within the body. Many of the postures are named after animals (such as the dog, peacock, pigeon, crow and camel) or famous sages. The profound insight of Pattabhi Jois was his arrangement of postures into series that systematically stretch all of the important muscles in the body.

It is well known that there is an intimate connection between the way one breathes and one's mental and physical state. A person with a disciplined body will generally find it much easier to sit still for a deep meditation practice. Through the effort and discipline of yoga the practitioner gradually gains mastery over the fluctuations of the mind, and through postural practice keeps the body strong and flexible. Therein lies the goal of yoga, a practice that has developed in its different forms over many centuries, to facilitate freedom from the afflictions of the world, at the very least to a certain degree.

Dr Matthew Clark, Research Associate at SOAS University of London

Sun Salutation A & B

Sūrya Namaskāra A & B

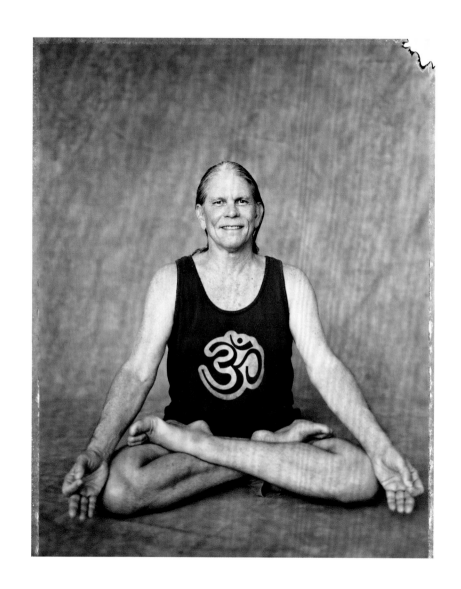

David Williams

The extroverted inward

To master the body
A way to shape emotions
To control the movements
A way to channel feelings

Self-awareness is of need
To be aware of anyone
Navigated by the heart
To cultivate the inner grace

A self-critic by nature
Comments of the mind
Challenging experiences
Teachers of the soul

A ray of light
Shines on the innermost
When outside's form
Gives grace and harmony

Insisting on freedom
The unique path to peace
Flood light to every corner
It is stillness of the mind

Samasthitiḥ

समस्थितिः

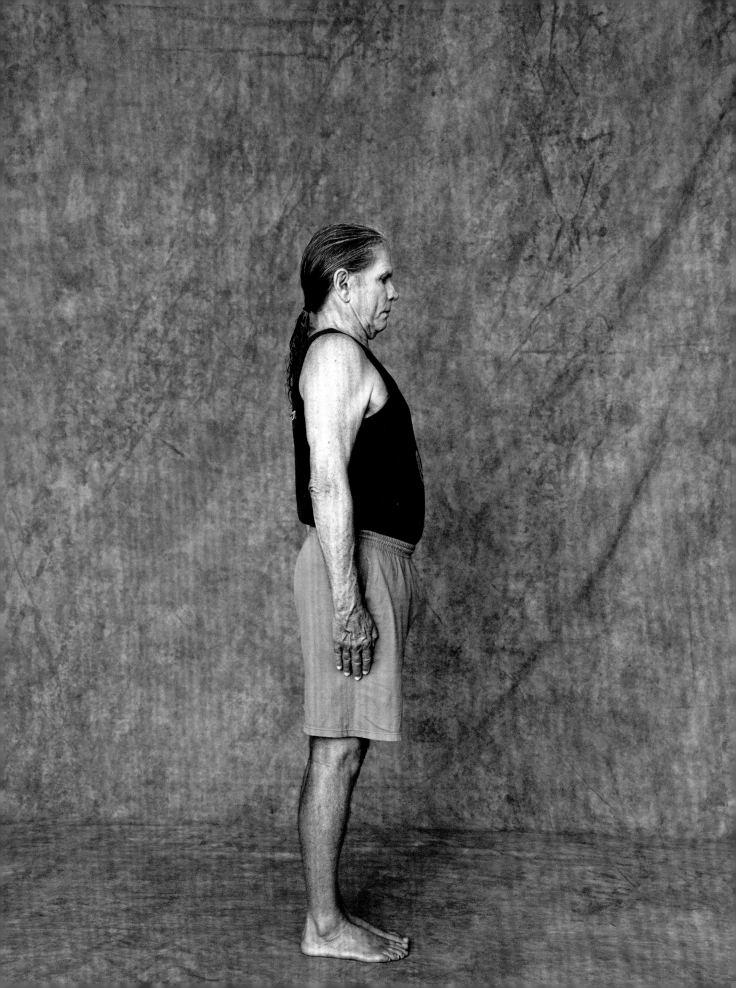

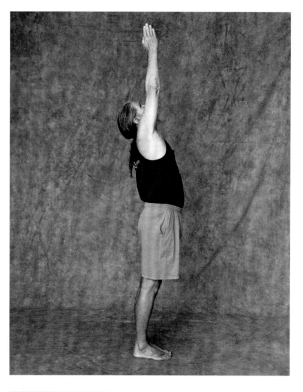

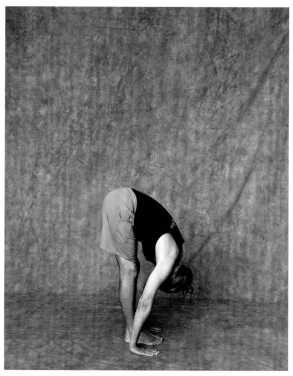

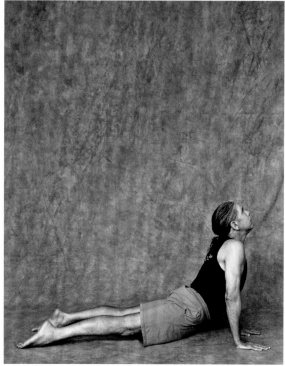

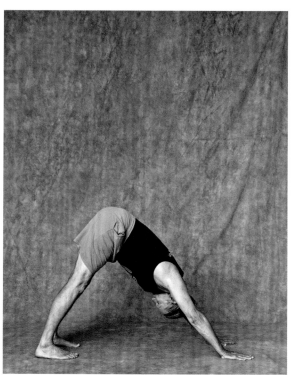

∧

Ūrdhva Vṛkṣāsana

ऊर्ध्ववृक्षासन

∨

Ūrdhva Mukha Śvānāsana

ऊर्ध्वमुखश्वानासन

∧

Uttānāsana A

उत्तानासन १

∨

Adho Mukha Śvānāsana

अधोमुखश्वानासन

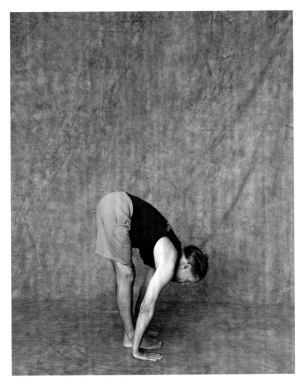

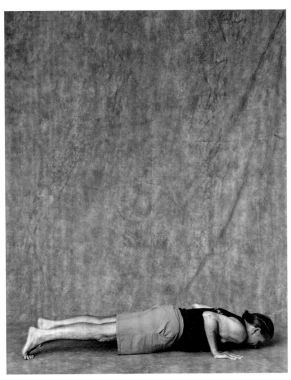

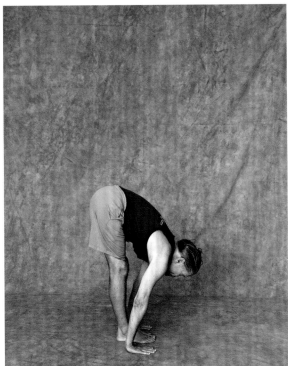

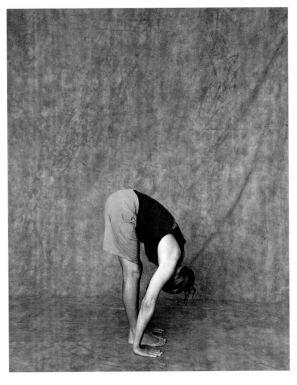

∧

Uttānāsana B

उत्तानासन २

∨

Uttānāsana B

उत्तानासन २

∧

Caturāṅga Daṇḍāsana

चतुरङ्गदण्डासन

∨

Uttānāsana A

उत्तानासन १

23

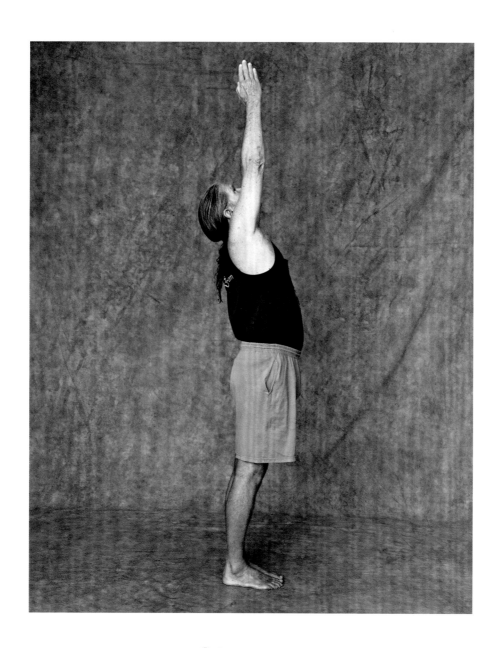

Ūrdhva Vṛkṣāsana

ऊर्ध्ववृक्षासन

>

Samasthitiḥ

समस्थितिः

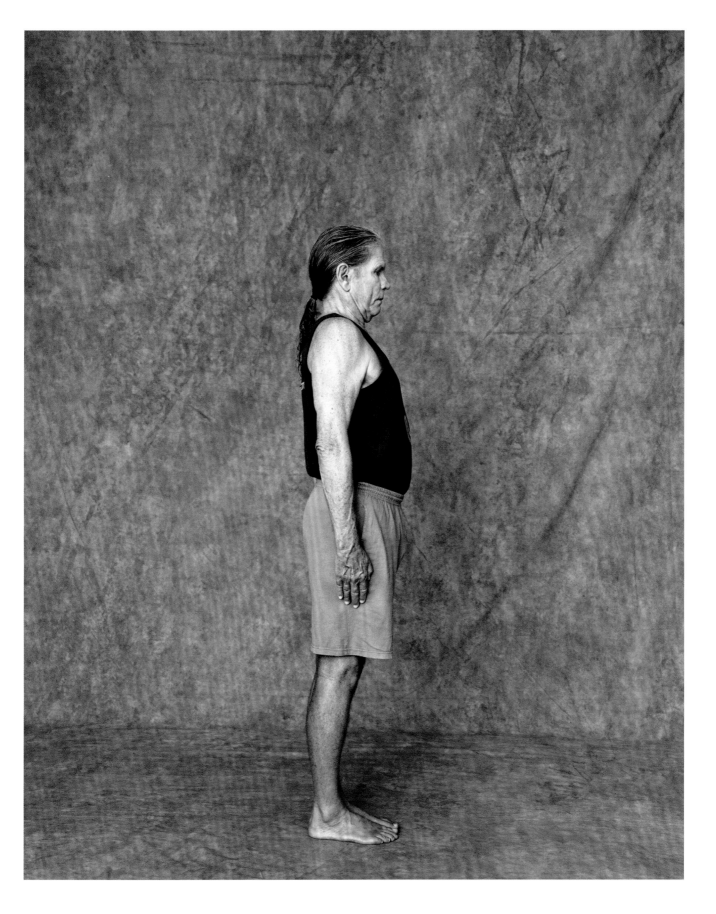

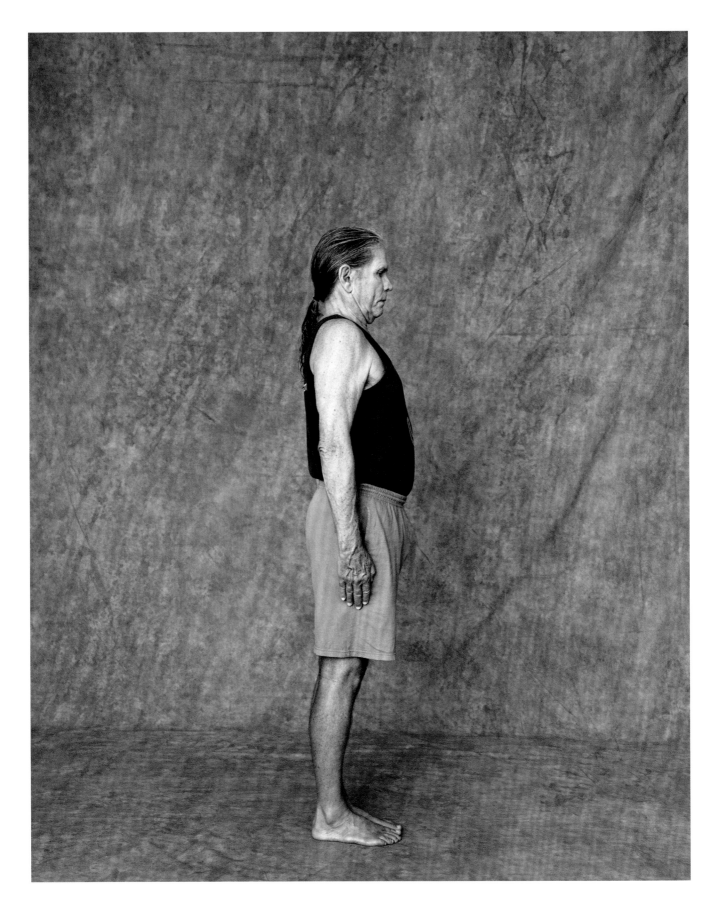

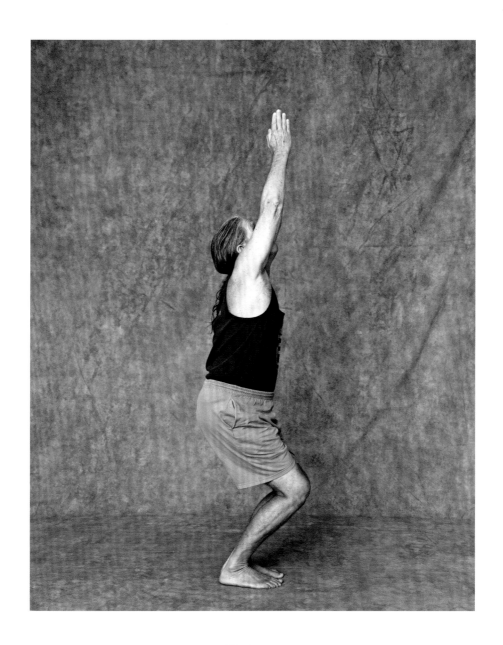

Utkaṭāsana

उत्कटासन

<

Samasthitiḥ

समस्थितिः

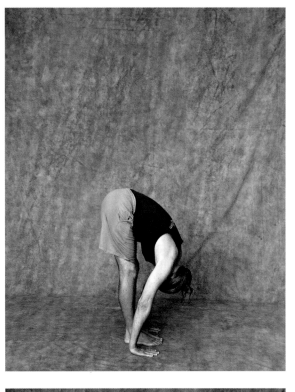

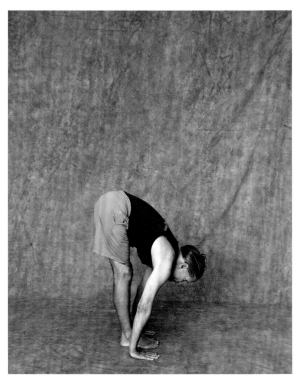

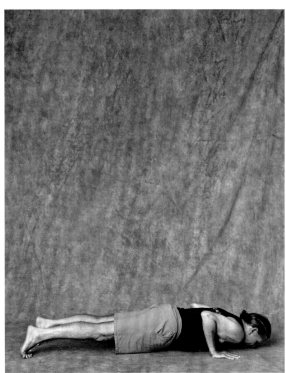

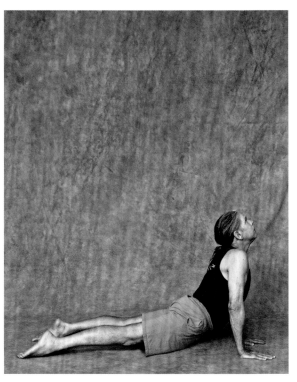

∧

Uttānāsana A

उत्तानासन १

∨

Caturāṅga Daṇḍāsana

चतुराङ्गदण्डासन

∧

Uttānāsana B

उत्तानासन २

∨

Ūrdhva Mukha Śvānāsana

ऊर्ध्वमुखश्वानासन

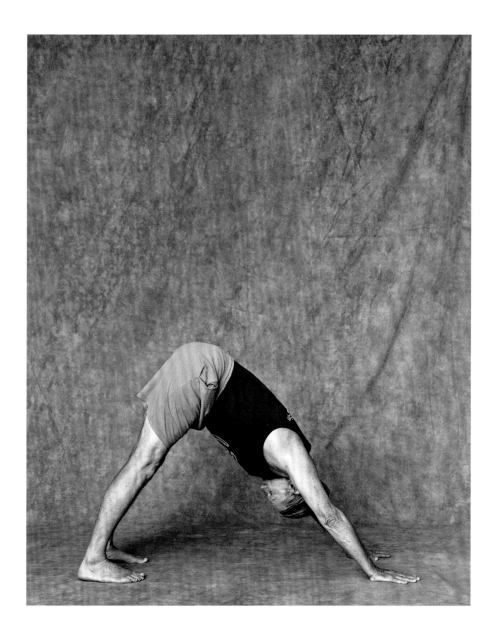

Adho Mukha Śvānāsana

अधोमुखश्वानासन

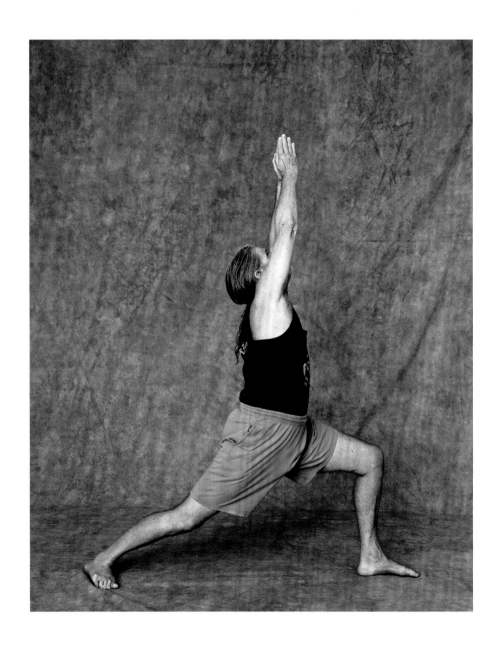

Vīrabhadrāsana

वीरभद्रासन

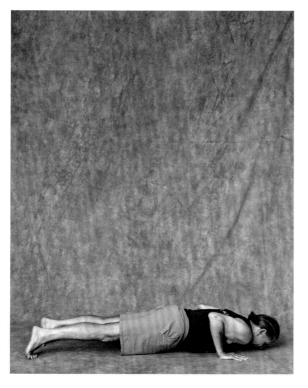

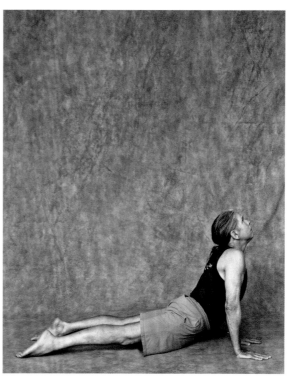

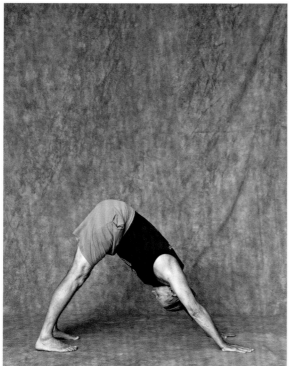

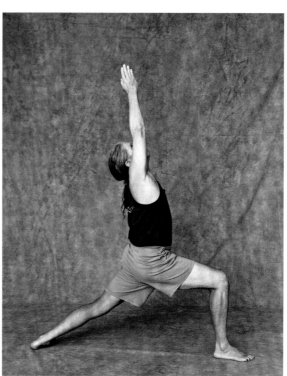

∧

Caturāṅga Daṇḍāsana

चतुरङ्गदण्डासन

∨

Adho Mukha Śvānāsana

अधोमुखश्वानासन

∧

Ūrdhva Mukha Śvānāsana

ऊर्ध्वमुखश्वानासन

∨

Vīrabhadrāsana

वीरभद्रासन

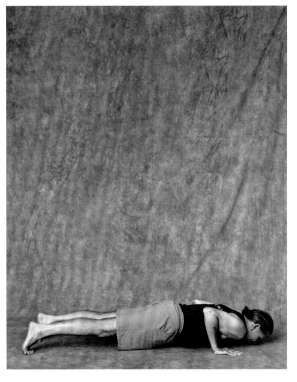

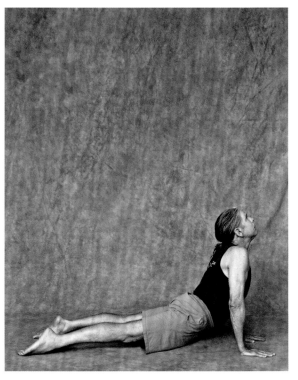

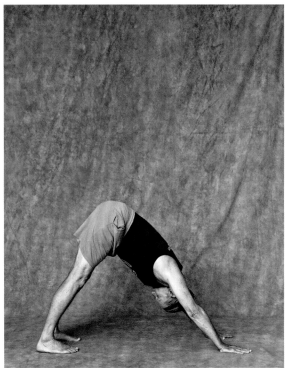

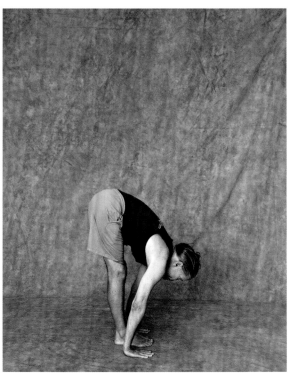

∧

Caturāṅga Daṇḍāsana

चतुराङ्गदण्डासन

∨

Adho Mukha Śvānāsana

अधोमुखश्वानासन

∧

Ūrdhva Mukha Śvānāsana

ऊर्ध्वमुखश्वानासन

∨

Uttānāsana B

उत्तानासन २

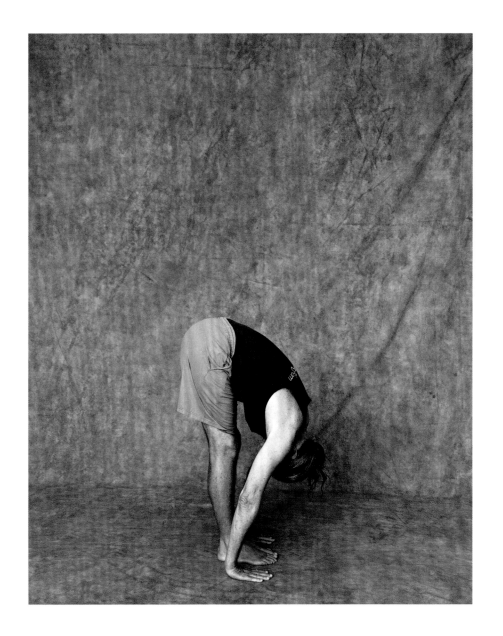

Uttānāsana A

उत्तानासन १

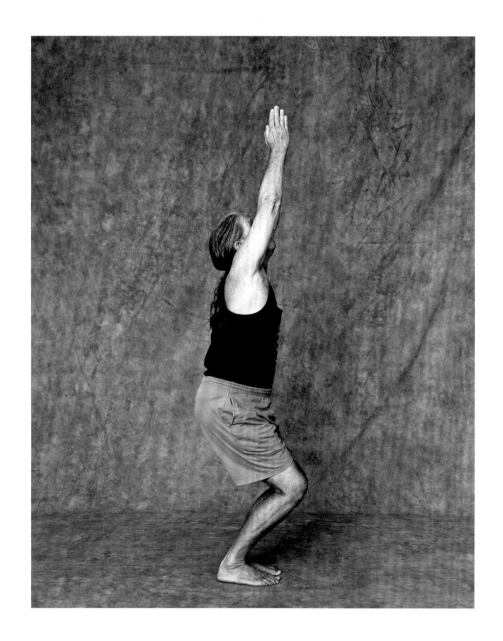

Utkaṭāsana

उत्कटासन

>

Samasthitiḥ

समस्थितिः

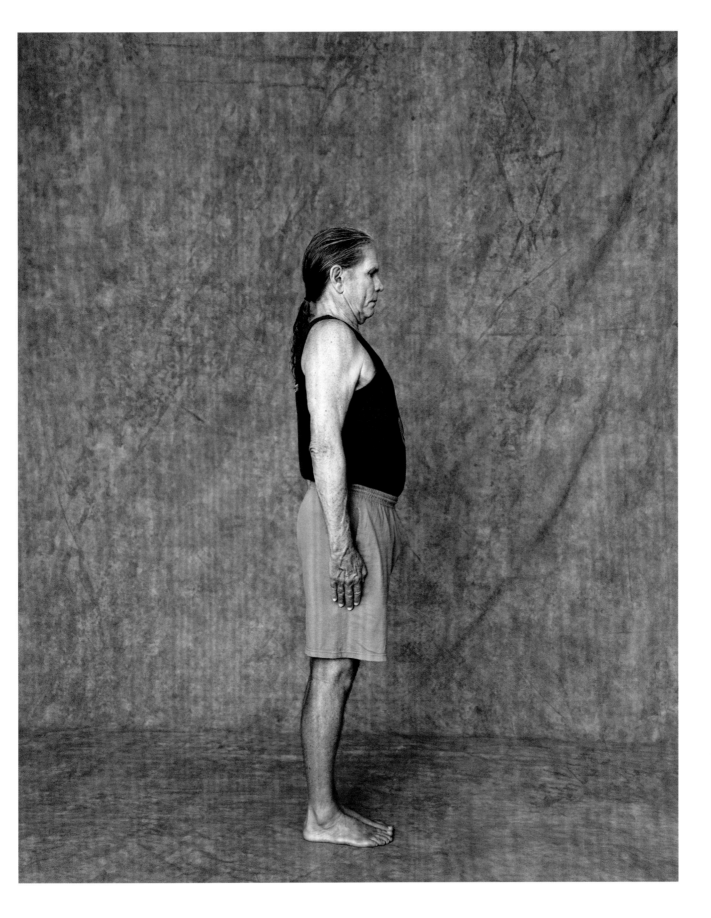

Fundamental Positions

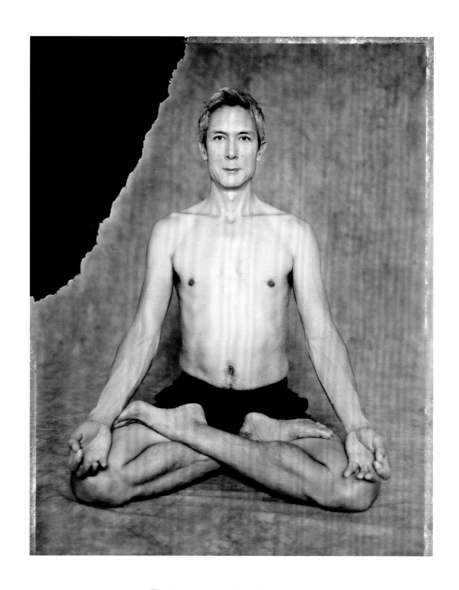

Gingi Lee

Blaze the trail
The inner restlessness
Where will it lead to?

Blaze the trail pathfinder
The adventurous spirit
Always ready for experiences

Blaze the trail initiator
The giving personality
Always wants to inspire others

Blaze the trail pioneer
The individual viewpoint
Always enjoying new projects

Variety can hide authenticity
Reflection is a strict teacher
Simplicity his greatest lesson

On slow feet
Feelings can't be hidden
The trailblazer to unlock hearts

Pādāṅguṣṭhāsana

पादाङ्गुष्ठासन

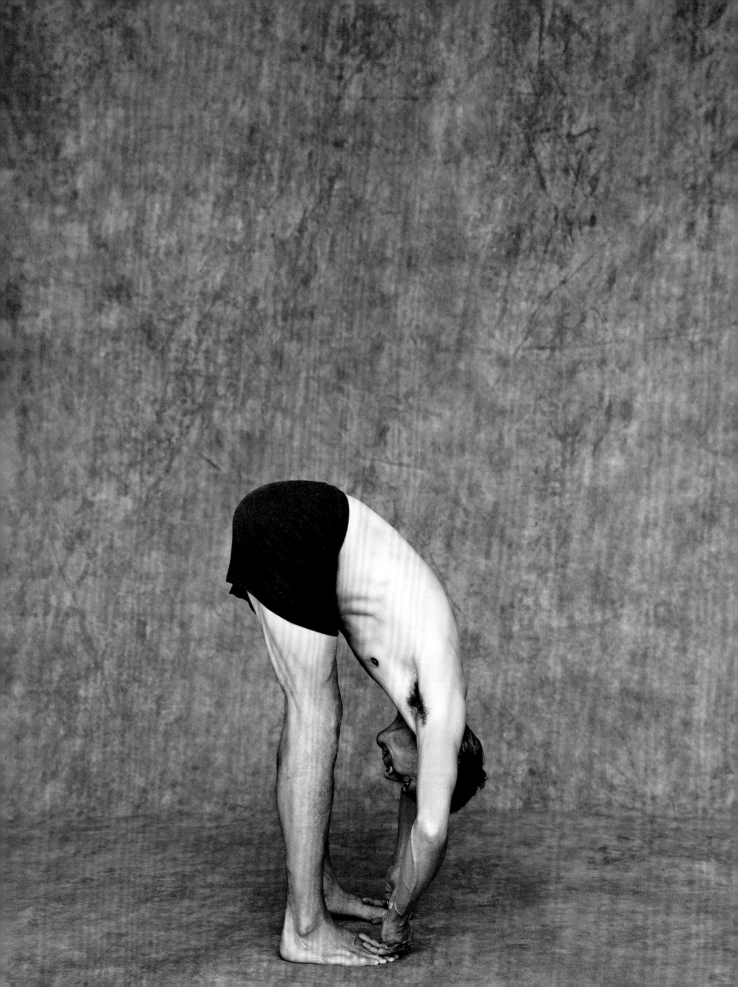

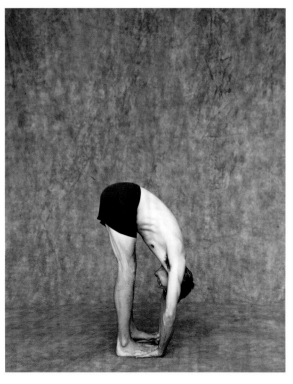

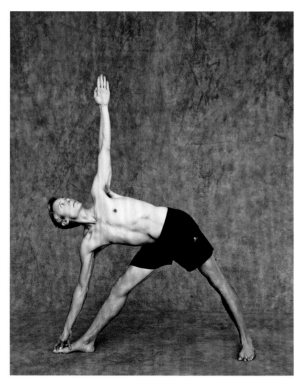

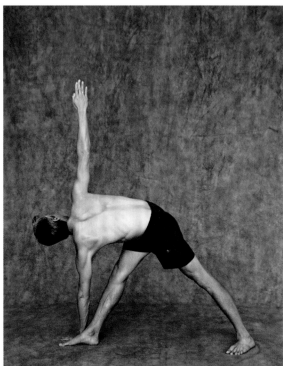

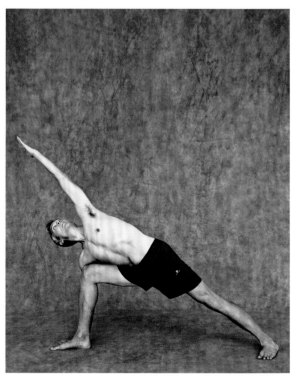

∧

Pāda Hastāsana

पादहस्तासन

∨

Parivṛtta Trikoṇāsana

उत्थितत्रिकोणासन

∧

Utthita Trikoṇāsana

उस्तिततिकोणासन

∨

Utthita Pārśva Koṇāsana

उत्थितपार्श्वकोणासन

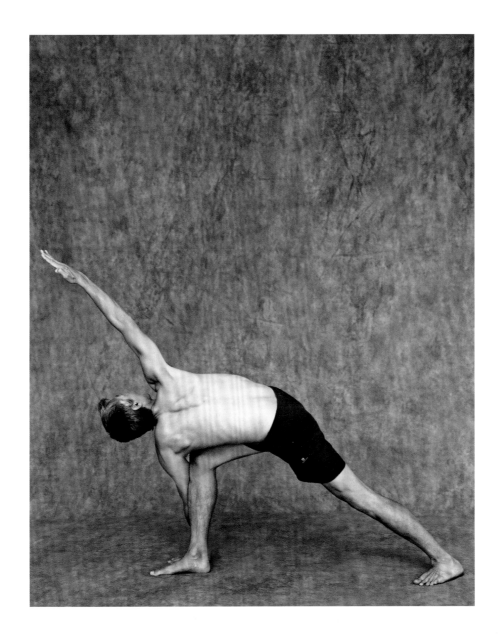

Parivṛtta Pārśva Koṇāsana

परिवृत्तपार्श्वकोणासन

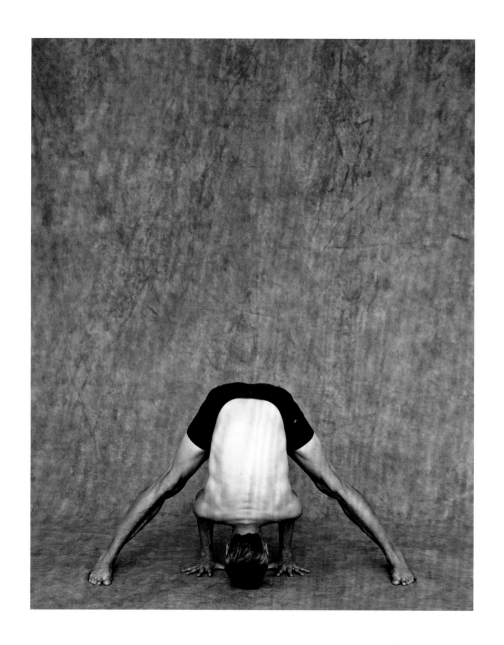

Prasārita Pādottānāsana A

प्रसारितपादोत्तानासन १

>

Prasārita Pādottānāsana B

प्रसारितपादोत्तानासन २

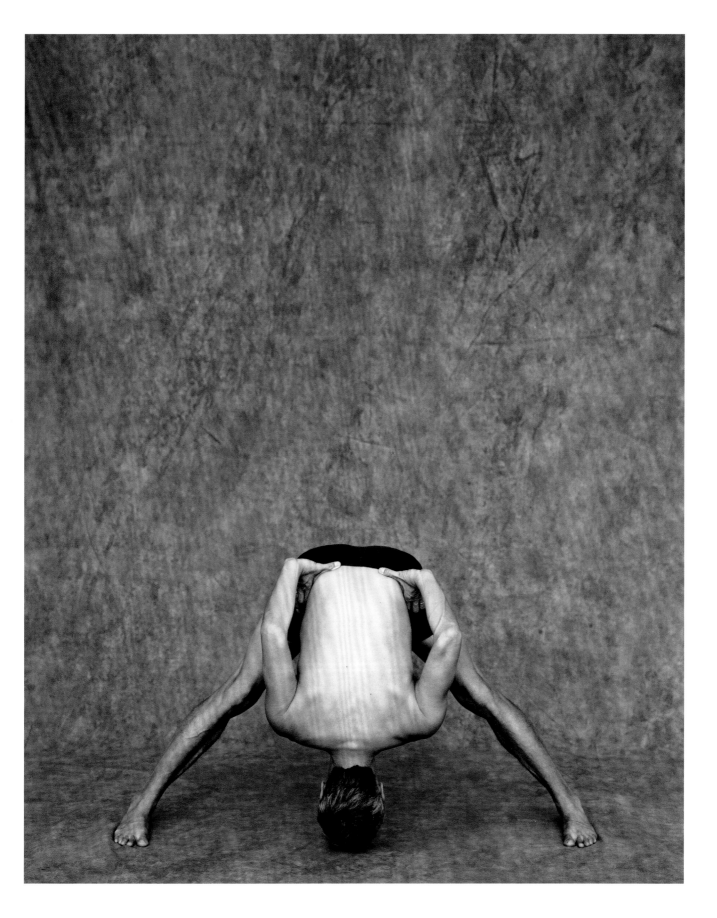

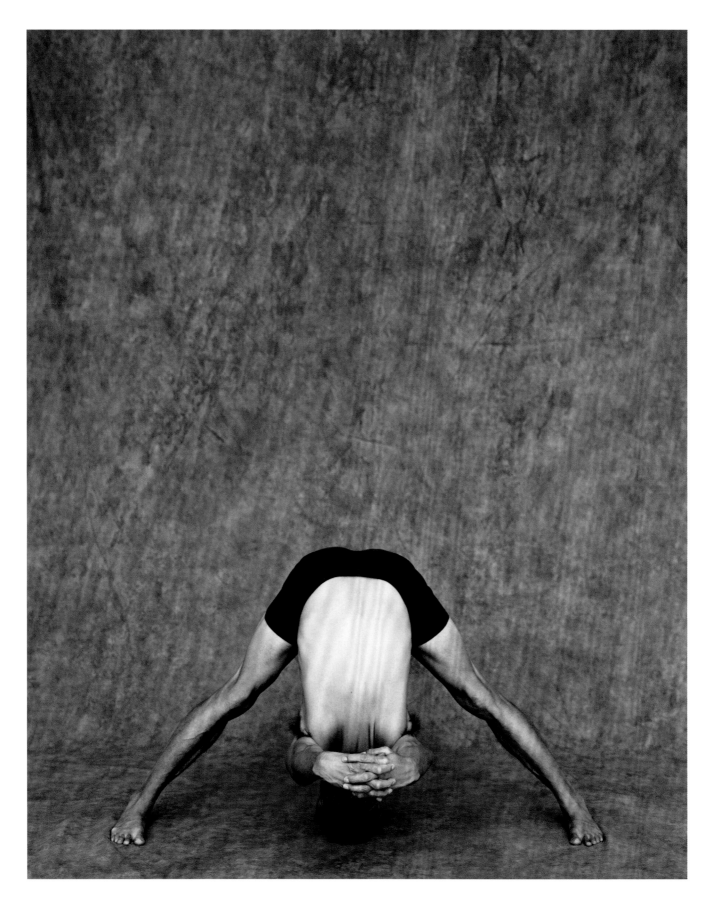

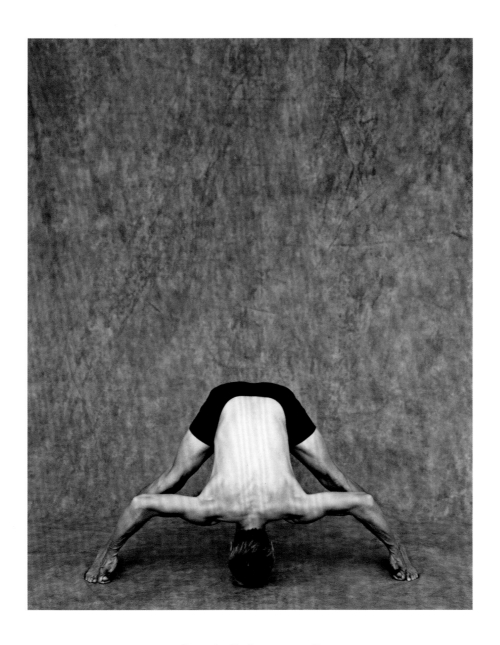

Prasārita Pādottānāsana D

प्रसारितपादोत्तानासन ८

Prasārita Pādottānāsana C

प्रसारितपादोत्तानासन ३

Pārśvottānāsana

पार्श्वोत्तानासन

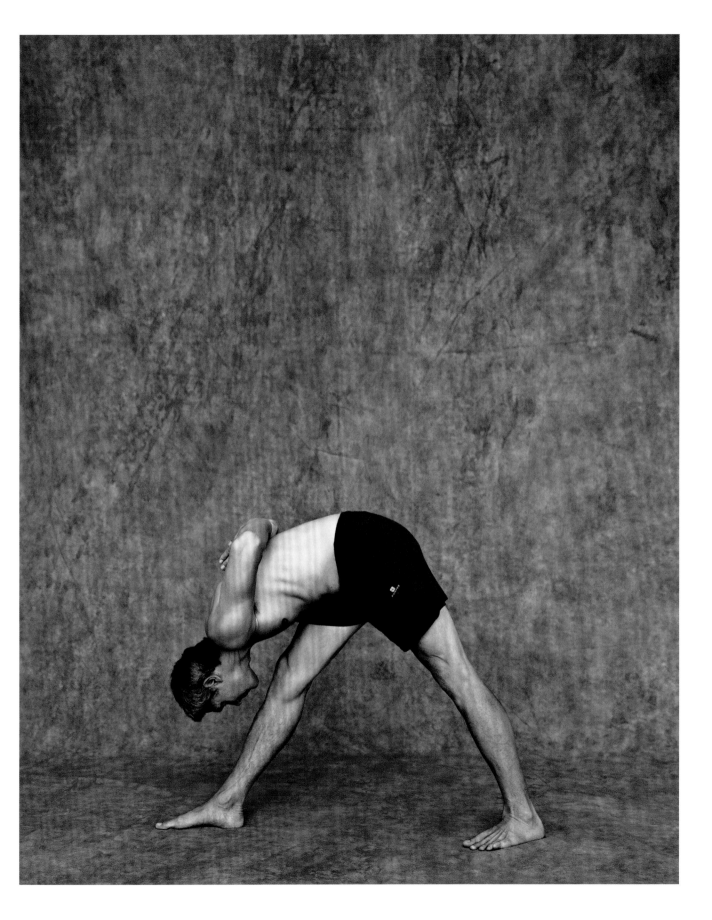

Primary

Yoga Cikitsā

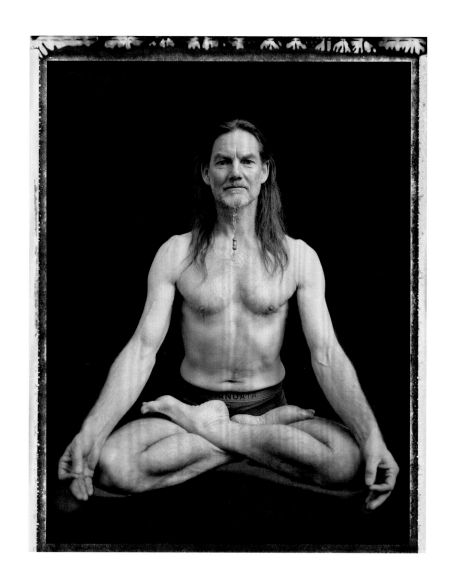

John Scott

I'm not judging
I'm pointing out the truth
My motivation is fair and just
The capability of piercing insight
It's clarity I offer

Thoughtful, responsible, stable

I'm not resting
I'm on an endless journey
Having a plan of action
Stimulating my sense of structure
It's to give shape and definition

Analytical, friendly, imaginative

I'm not giving up
I'm overcoming challenges
Success after early setbacks
Learn not be reactive nor secretive
It's a triumph over obstacles

Leading, sensitive, diplomatic

I'm testing myself
I'm guiding you
The objective evaluation
The good old common sense
The sudden flashes of inspiration

Intuitive, honourable, loyal

I'm learning from relationships
I'm growing with my defeats
Time filled with love
Fulfilment to be found here
My Essential Judgement

Utthita Hasta Pādāṅguṣṭhāsana A

उस्ततिहरतपादाङ्ग्षुारान १

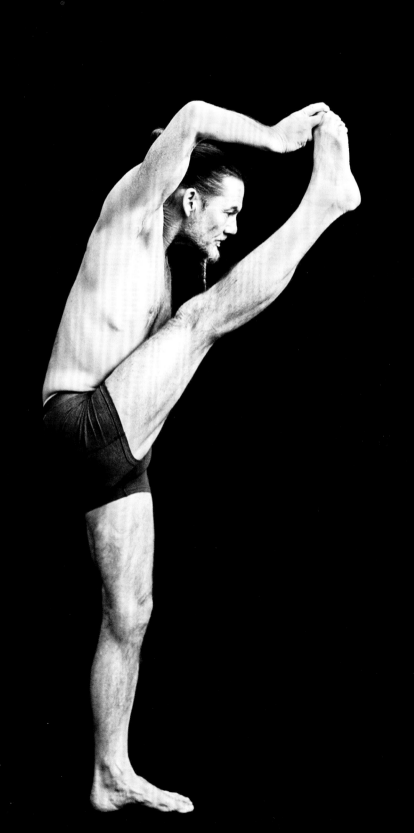

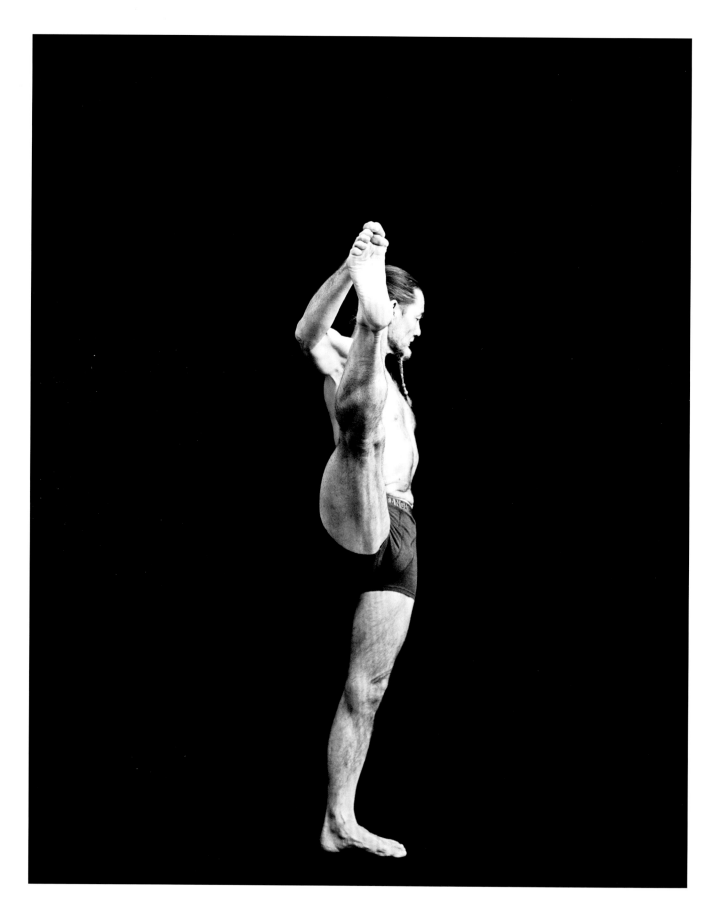

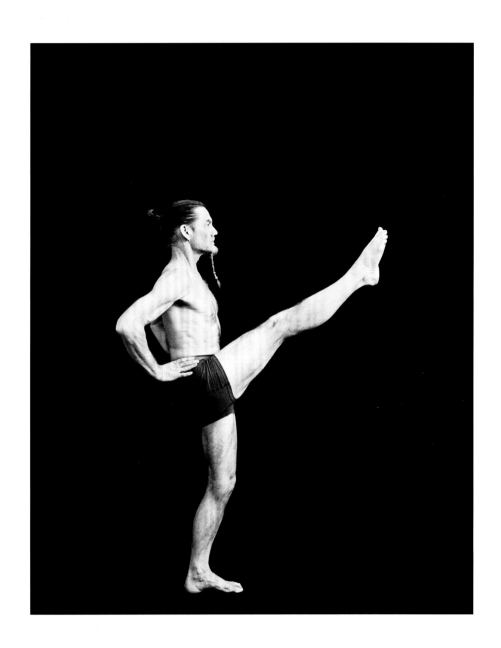

Utthita Hasta Pādāṅguṣṭhāsana B

उत्थितहस्तपादाङ्गुष्ठासन १

<

Utthita Pārśvasahita

उत्थितपार्श्वसहित

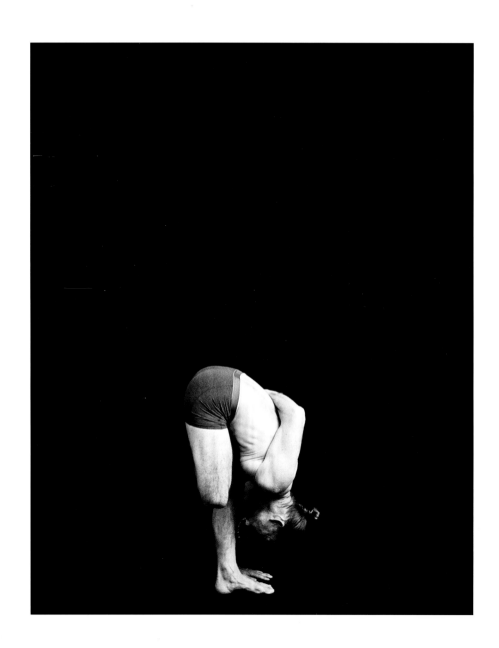

Ardha Baddha Padmottānāsana

अर्धबद्धपद्मोत्तानासन

>

Utkaṭāsana

उत्कटासन

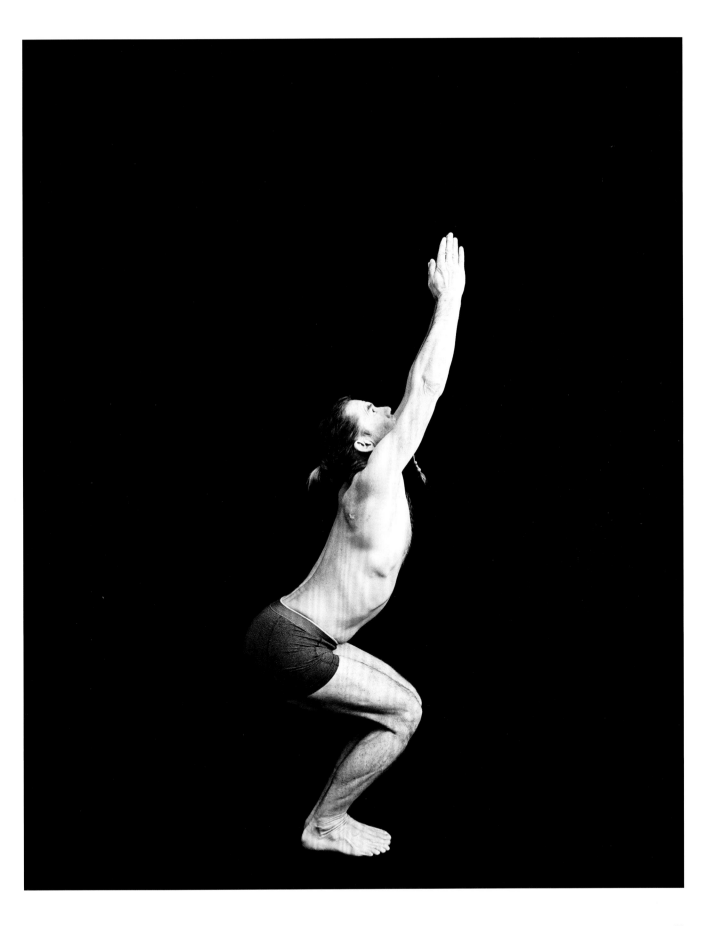

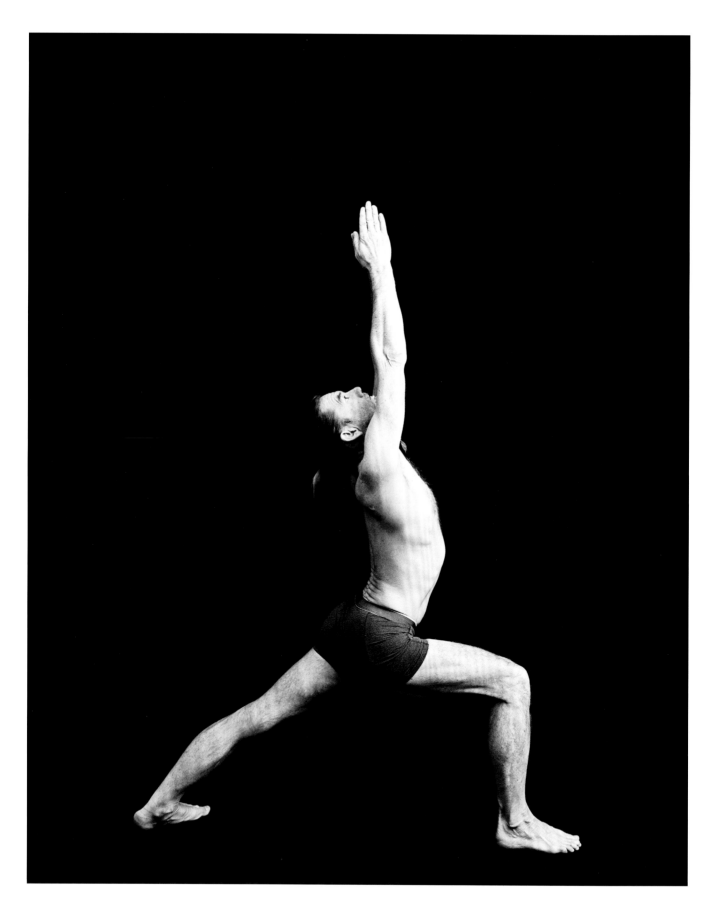

Vīrabhadrāsana A

वीरभद्रासन १

Vīrabhadrāsana B

वीरभद्रासन २

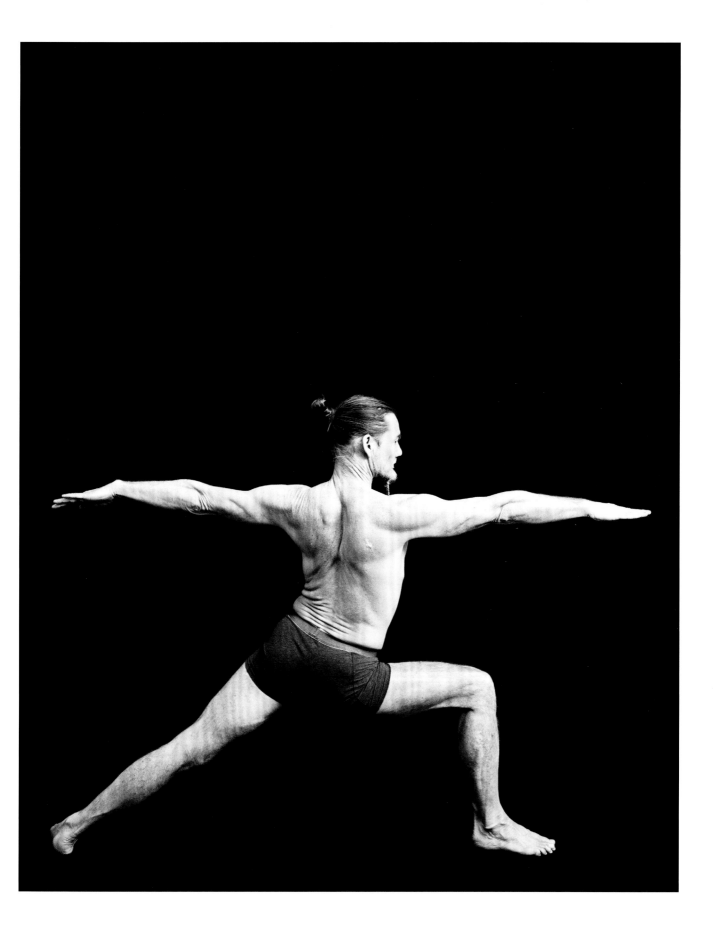

Daṇḍāsana

दण्डासन

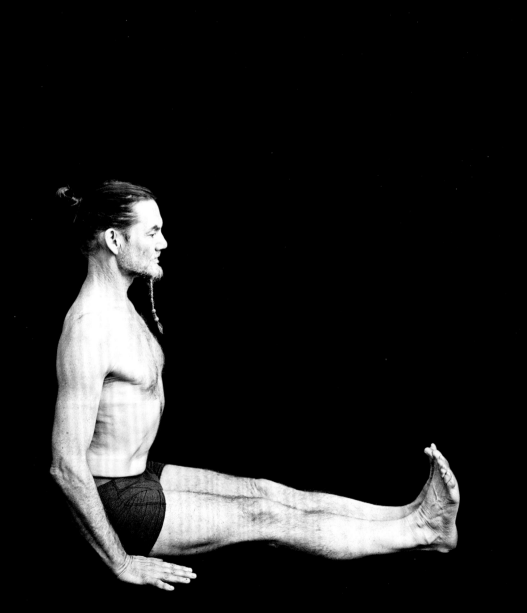

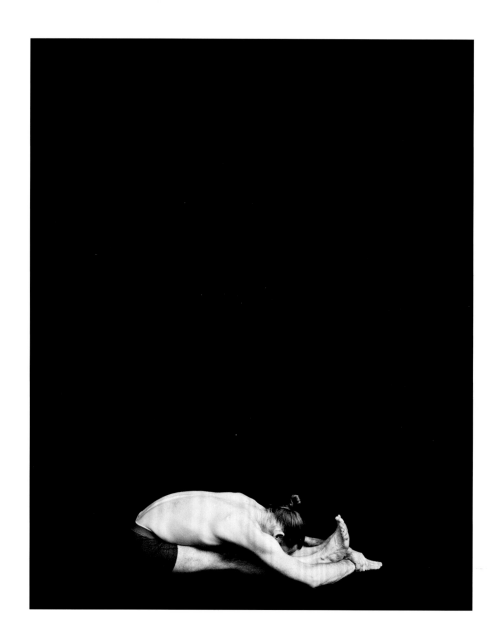

Paścimottānāsana

पश्चिमोत्तानासन

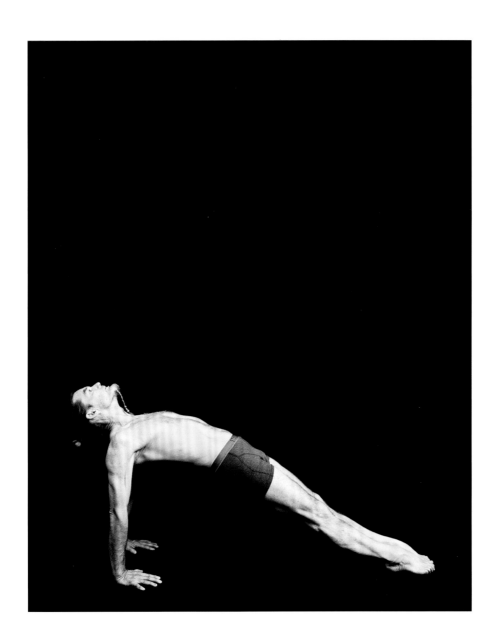

Pūrvottānāsana

पूर्वोत्तानासन

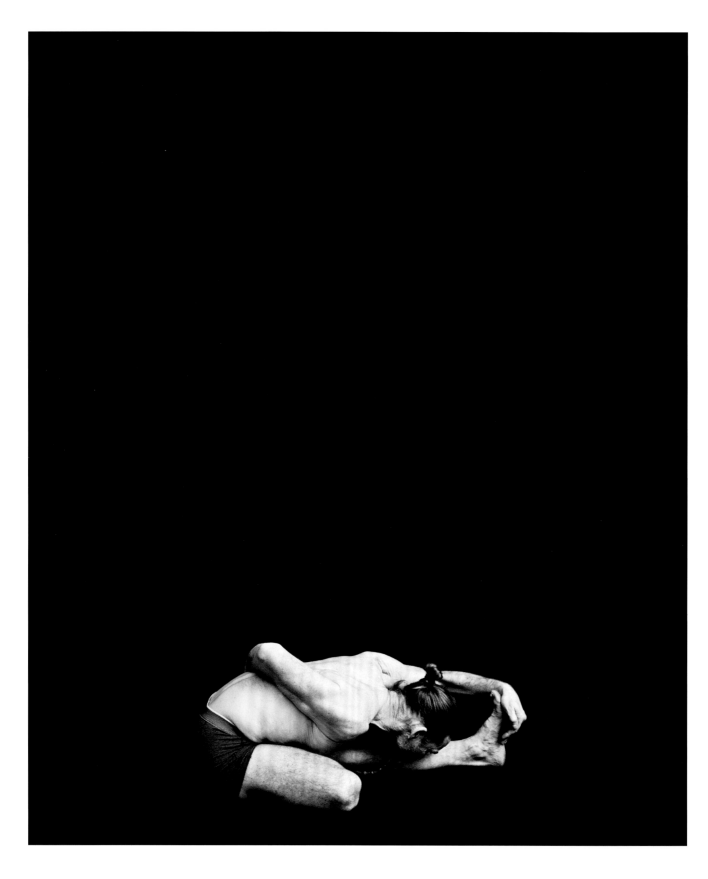

Ardha Baddha Padma Paścimottānāsana

अर्धबद्धपद्मपश्चिमोत्तानासन

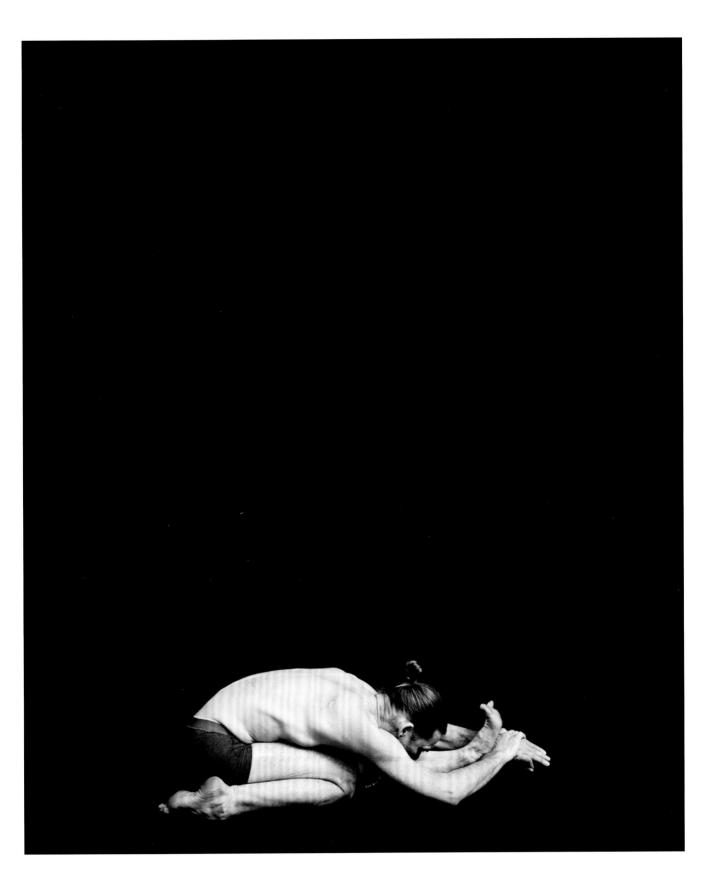

Tryaṅga Mukhaika Pāda Paścimottānāsana

त्र्यङ्गमुखैकपादपश्चिमोत्तानासन

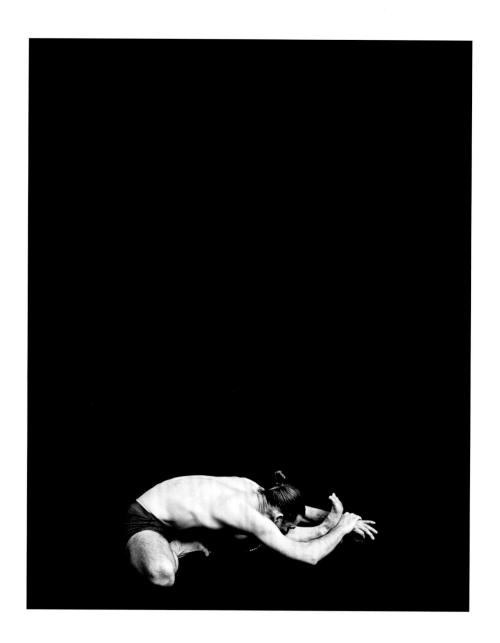

Jānu Śīrṣāsana A

जानुशीर्षासन १

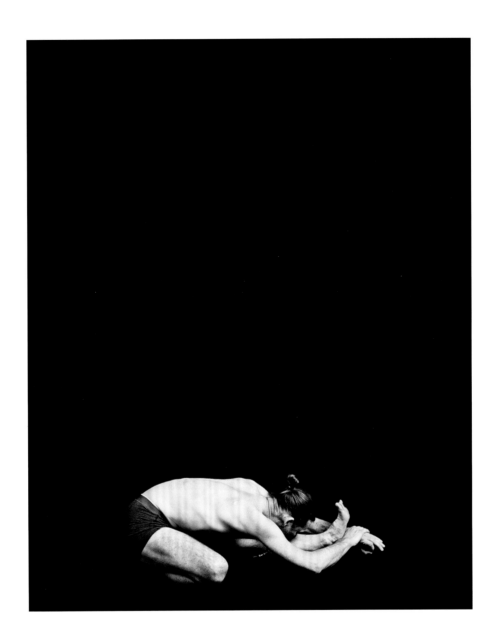

Jānu Śīrṣāsana B

जानुशीर्षासन २

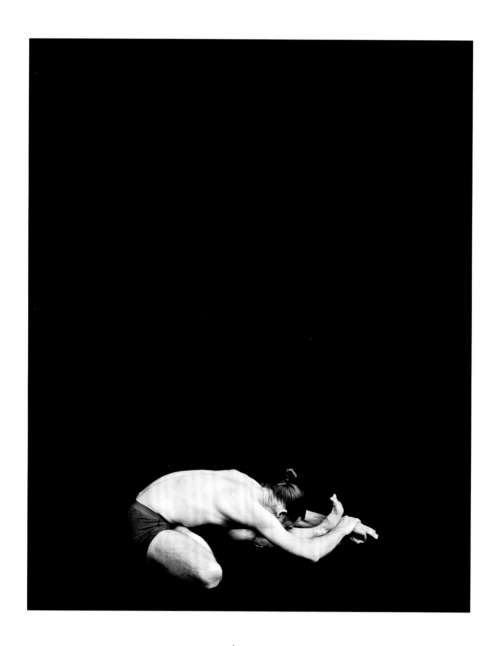

Jānu Śīrṣāsana C

जानुशीर्षासन ३

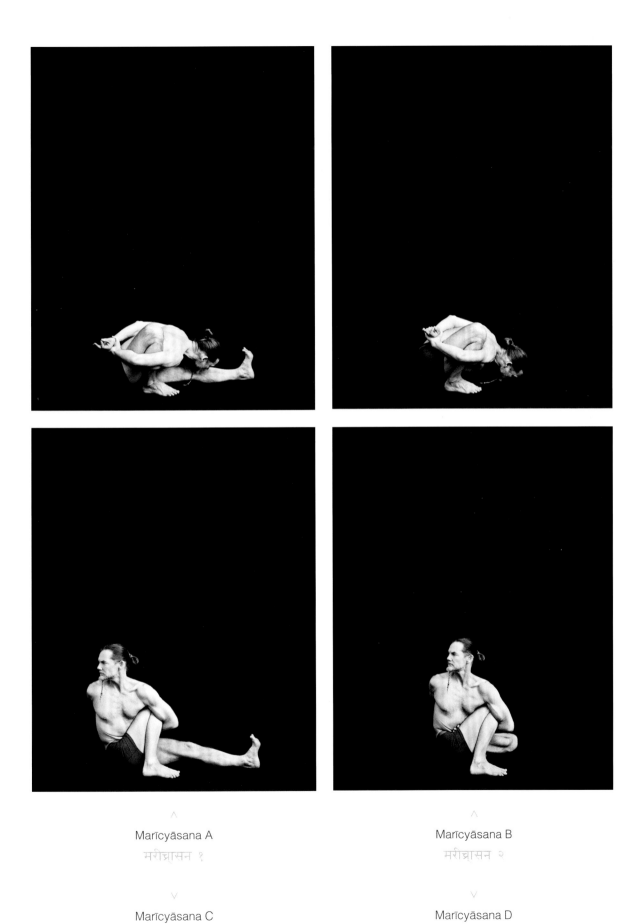

Marīcyāsana A

मरीच्यासन १

Marīcyāsana B

मरीच्यासन २

Marīcyāsana C

मरीच्यासन ३

Marīcyāsana D

मरीच्यासन ४

Nāvāsana

नावासन

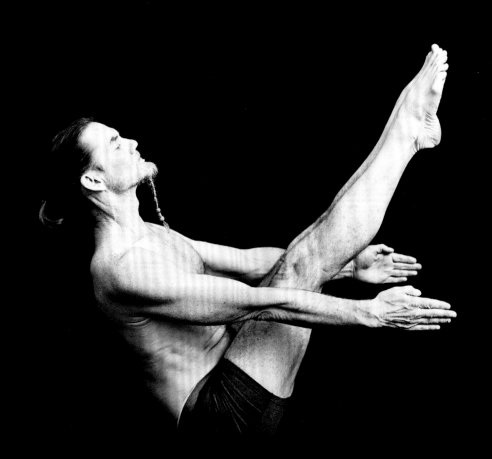

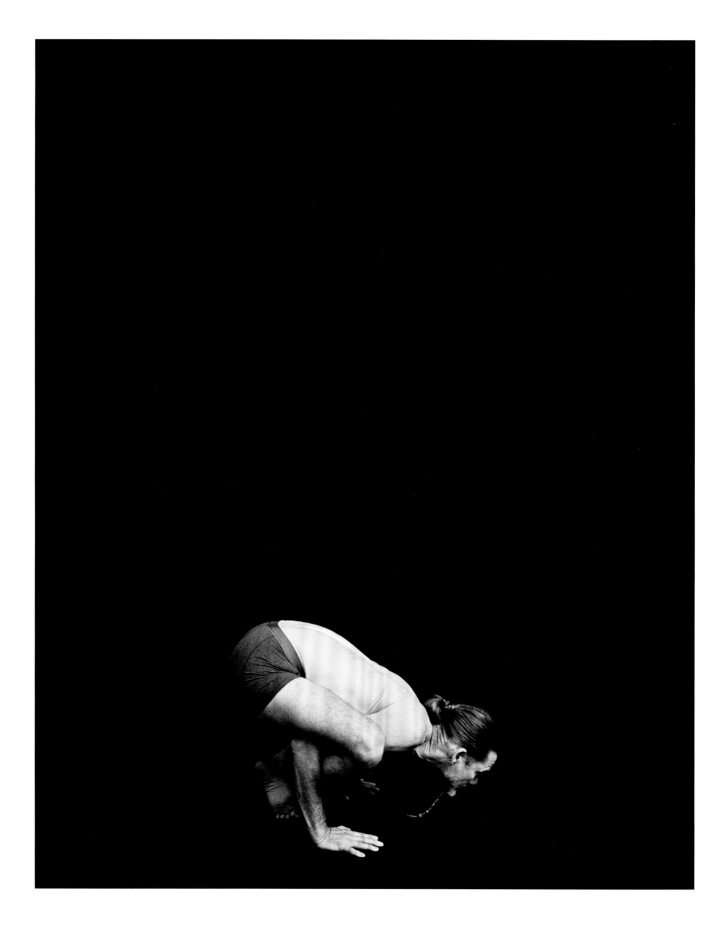

Bhuja Pīḍāsana

भुजपीडासन

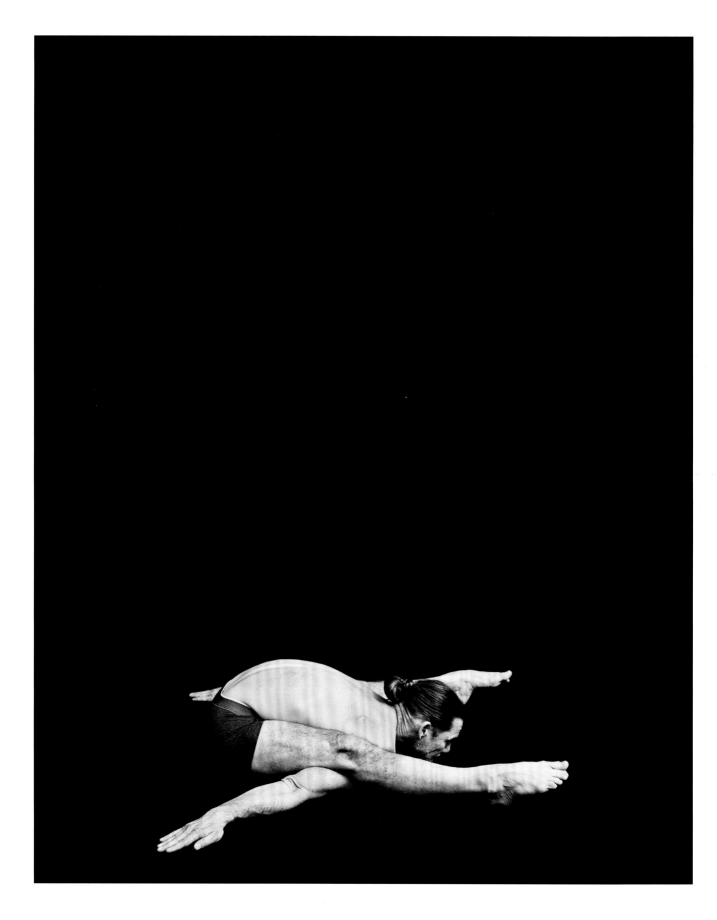

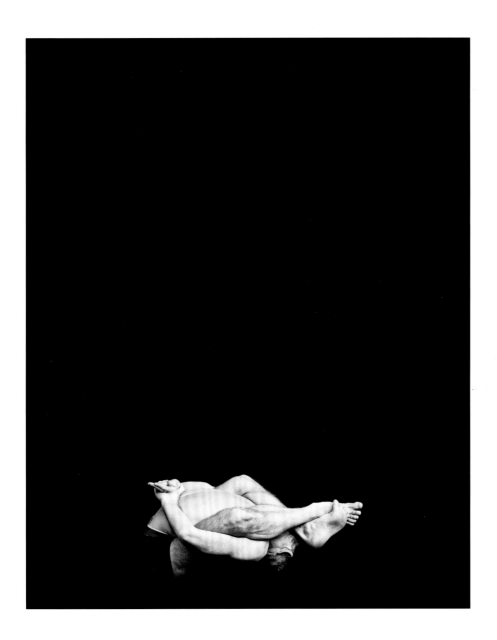

Supta Kūrmāsana

सुप्तकूर्मासन

<

Kūrmāsana

कूर्मासन

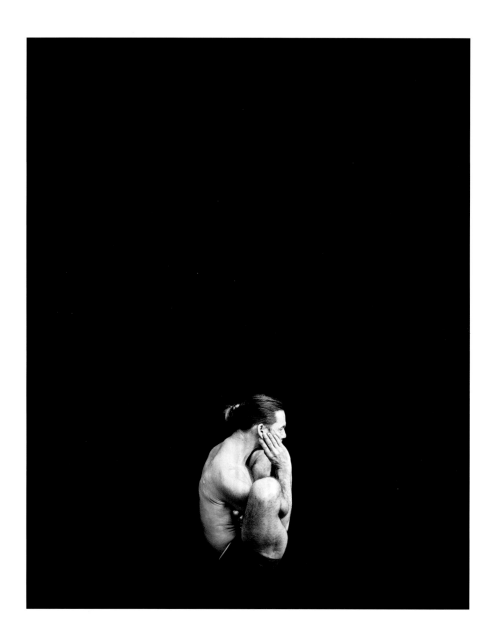

Garbha Piṇḍāsana

गर्भपिण्डासन

>

Kukkuṭāsana

कुक्कुटासन

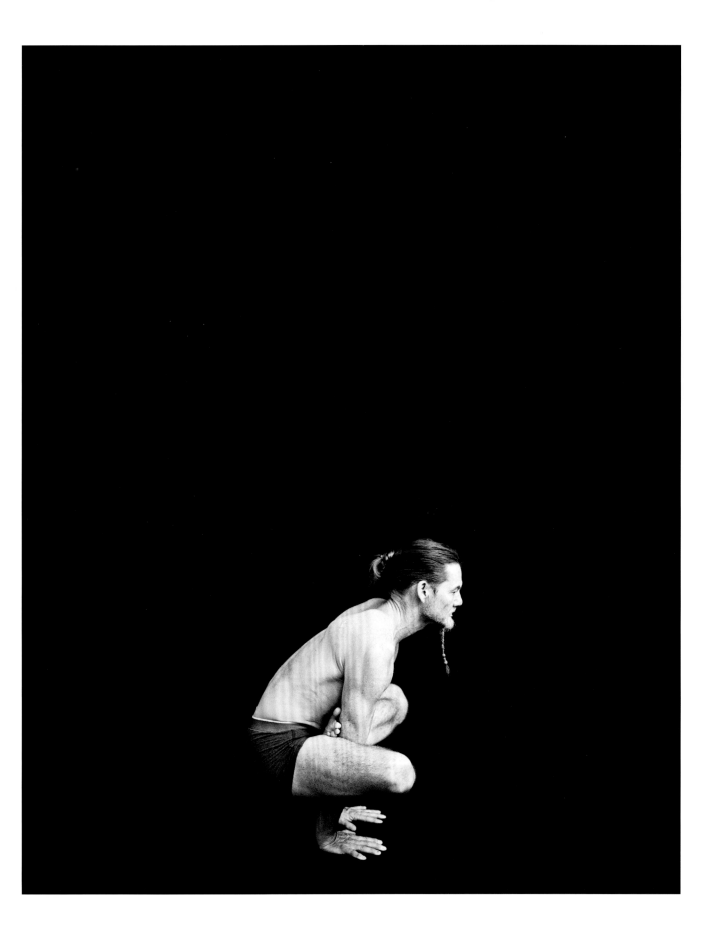

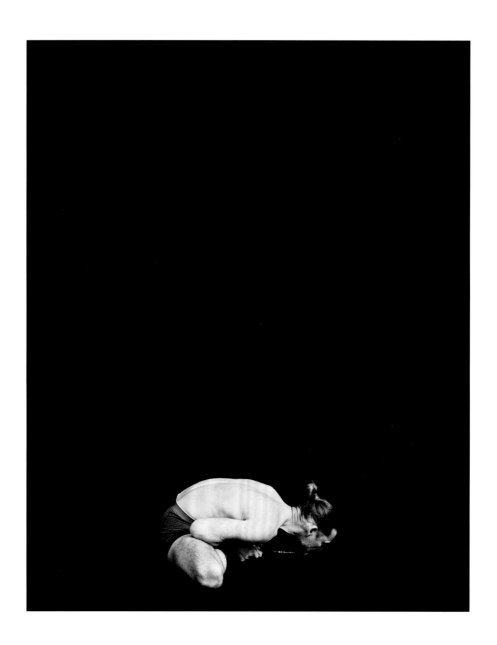

Baddha Koṇāsana A

बद्धकोणासन १

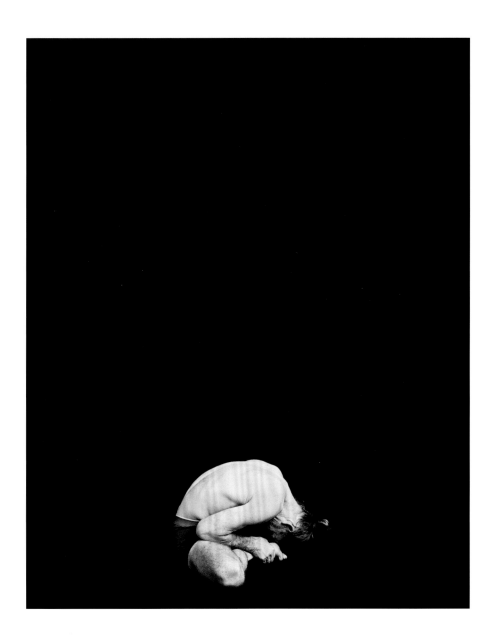

Baddha Koṇāsana B

बद्धकोणासन २

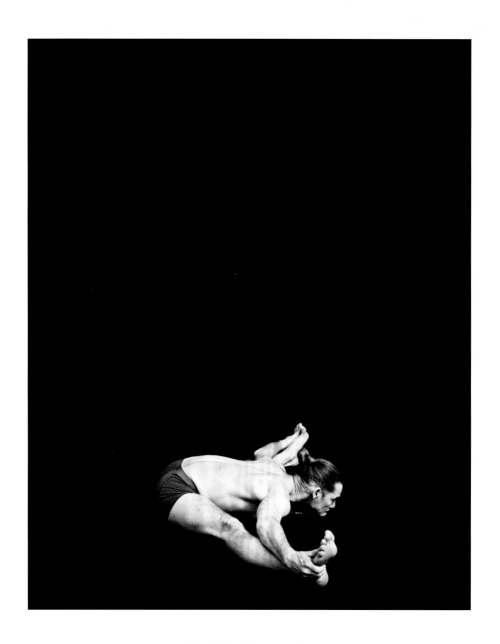

Upaviṣṭha Koṇāsana A

उपविष्ठकोणासन १

>

Upaviṣṭha Koṇāsana B

उपविष्ठकोणासन २

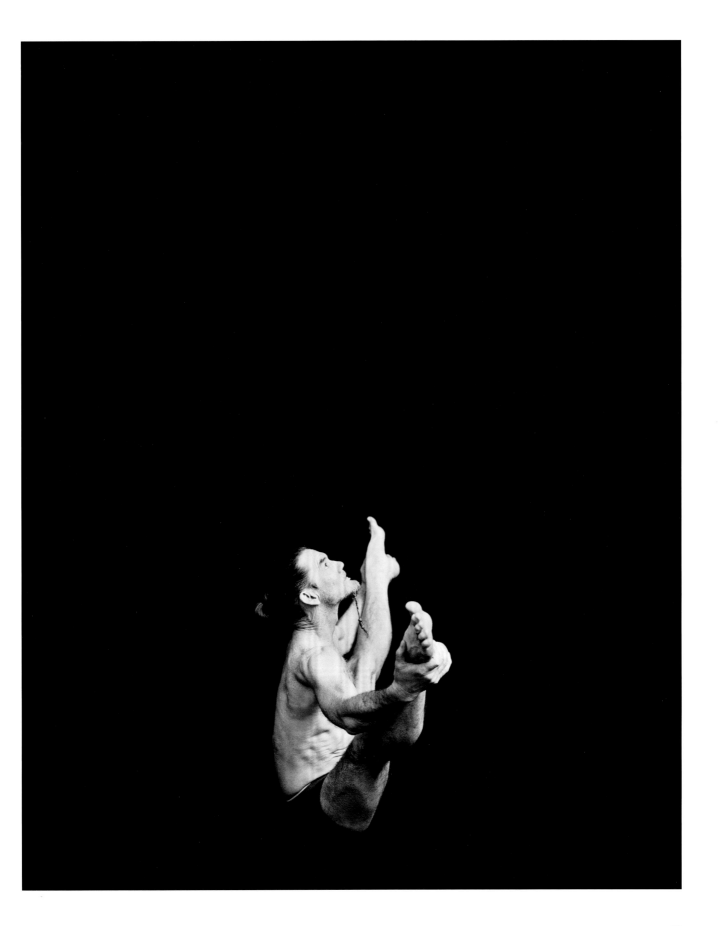

Supta Koṇāsana

सुप्तकोणासन

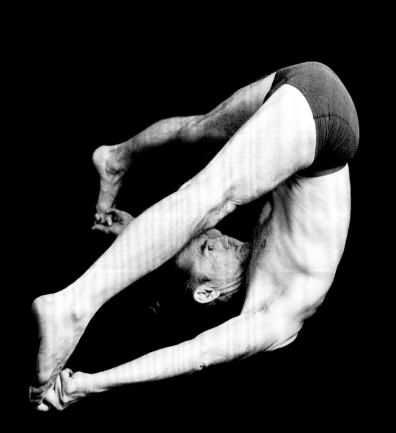

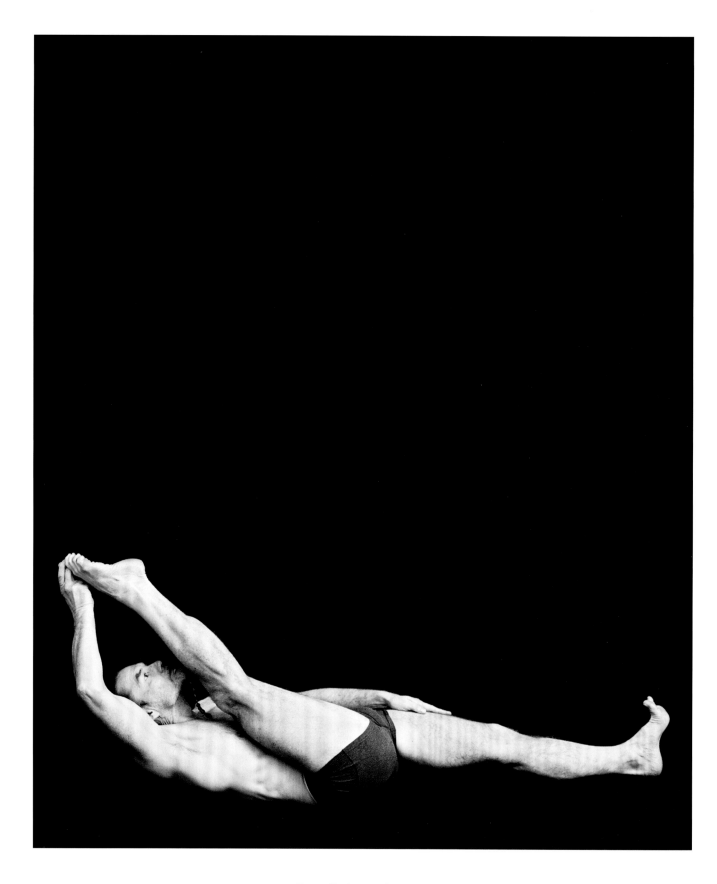

Supta Pādāṅguṣṭhāsana

सुप्तपादाङ्गुष्ठासन

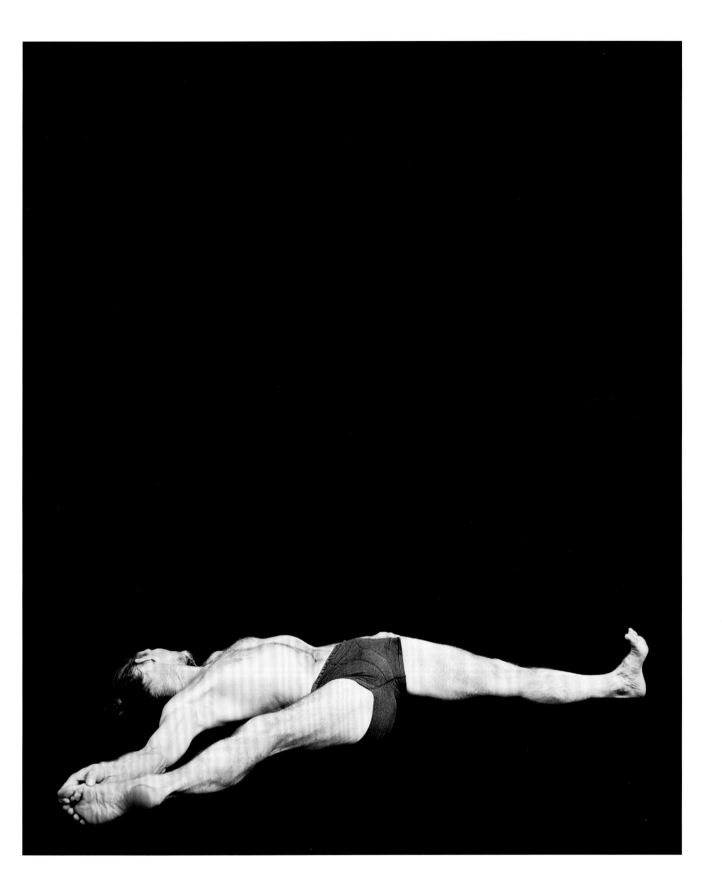

Supta Pārśvasahita

सुप्तपार्श्वसहित

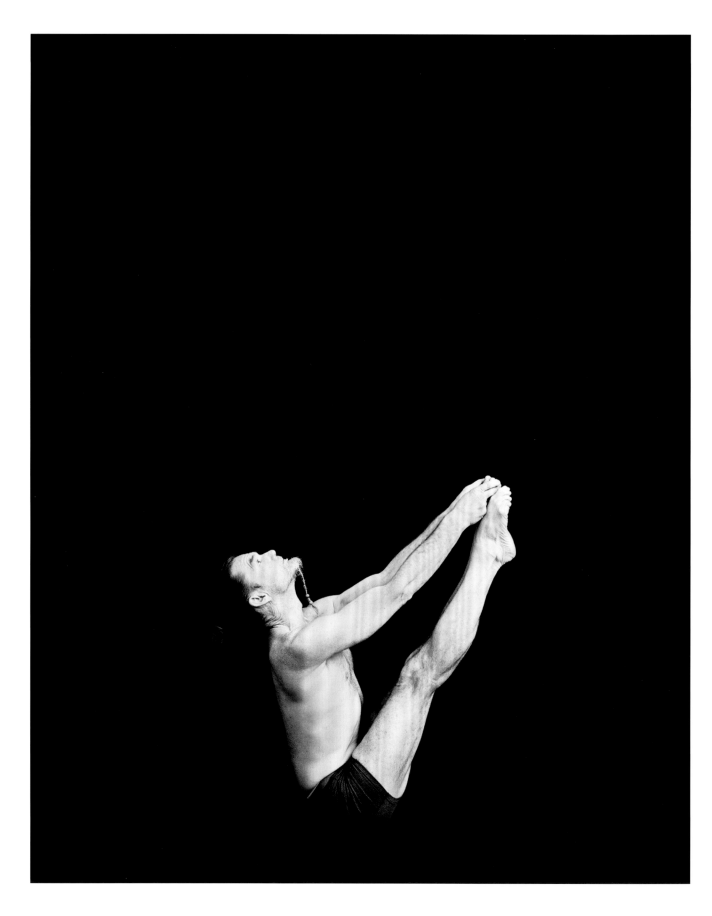

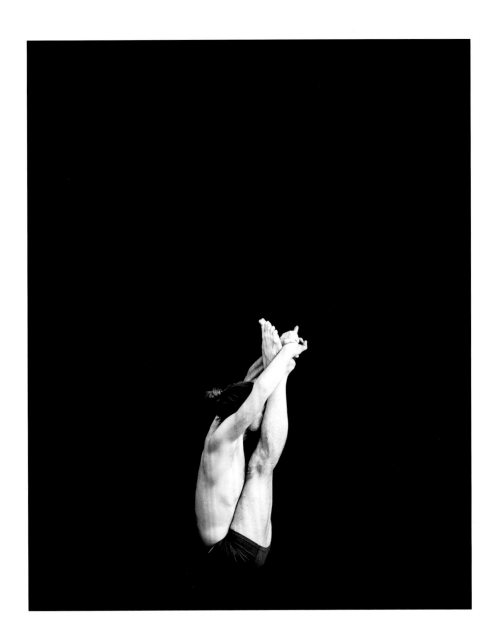

Ūrdhva Mukha Paścimottānāsana

ऊर्ध्वमुखपश्चिमोत्तानासन

Ubhaya Pādāṅguṣṭhāsana

उभयपादाङ्गुष्ठासन

Setu Bandhāsana

सेतुबन्धासन

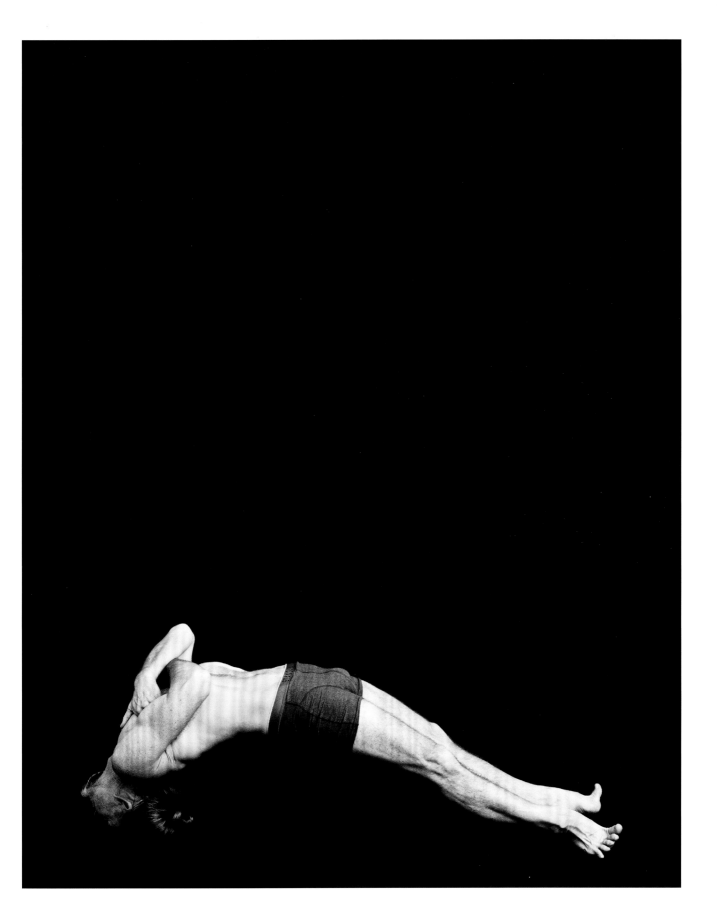

Ūrdhva Dhanurāsana

ऊर्ध्वधनुरासन

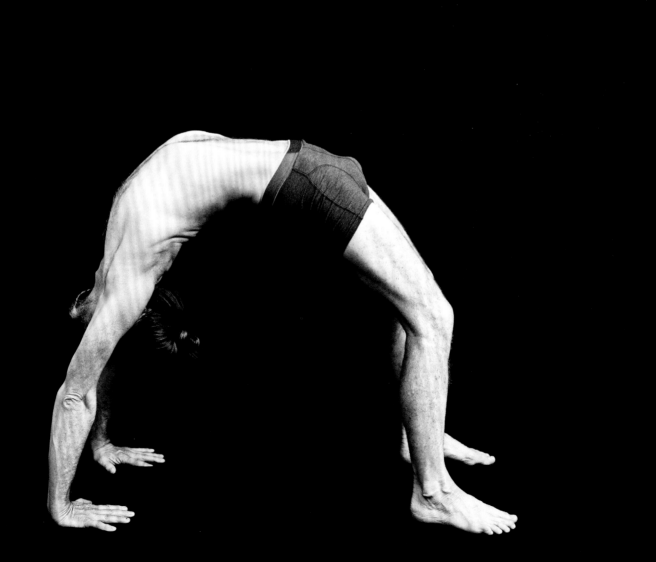

Intermediate

Nāḍi Śodhana

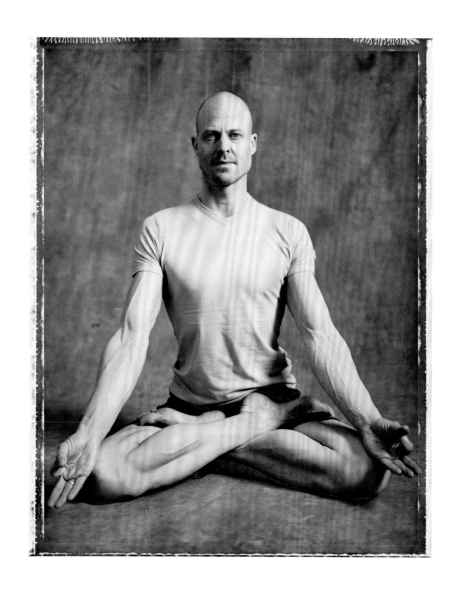

Ronald Steiner

Heart Thinks · Mind Feels · Body Speaks

Nothing more is possible
If it is only possible

What the head explores
Will reach the body
What the heart feels
The mind can never reach

Observe infinitely
Think deeply
Analyse sharply
Perform clearly

Sensitivity for others
Few words about the I
Patient, the warm heart
Peaceful, the cool mind

Everything is possible
When it seems impossible

Pāśāsana

पाशासन

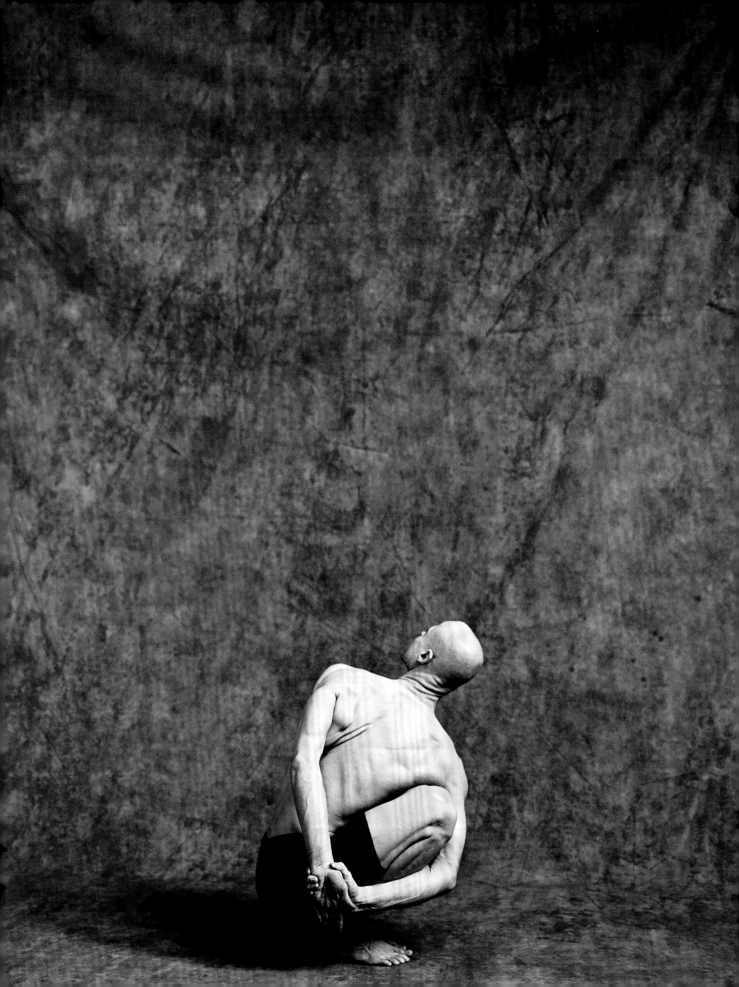

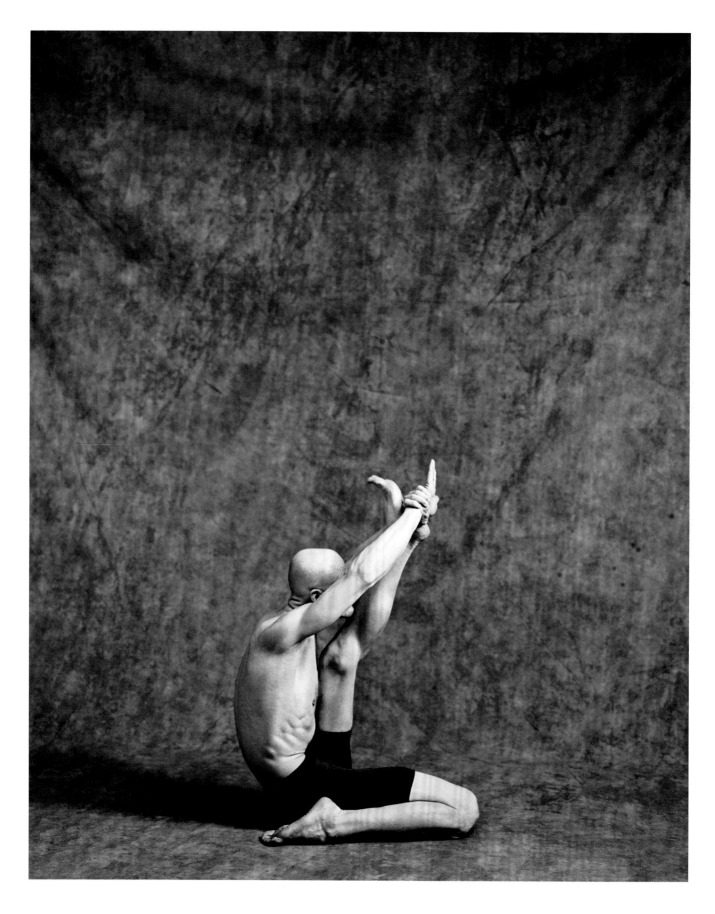

Krauñcāsana

कौश्चासन

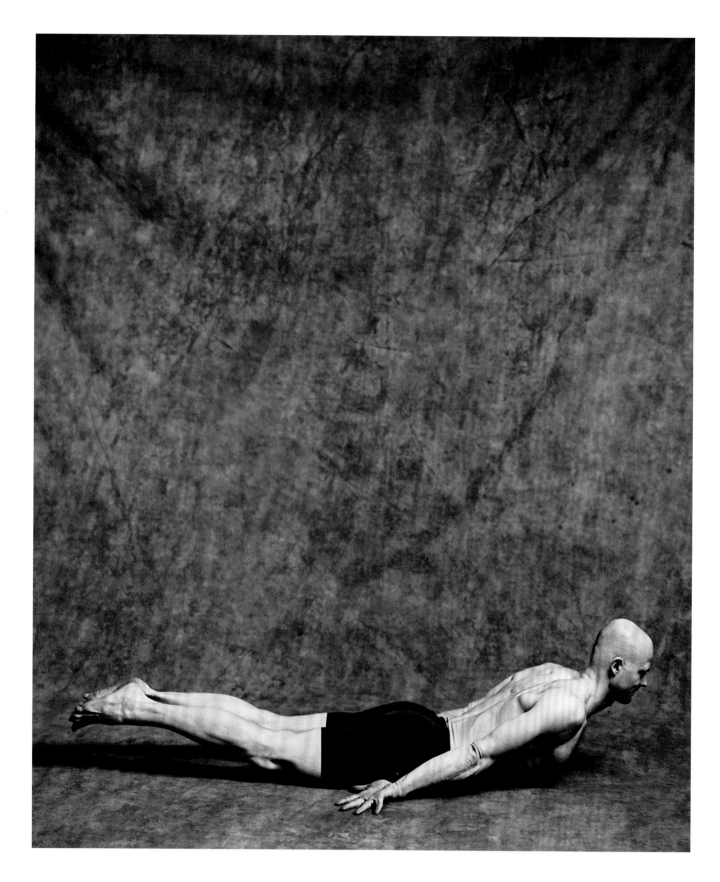

Śalabhāsana A

शलभासन १

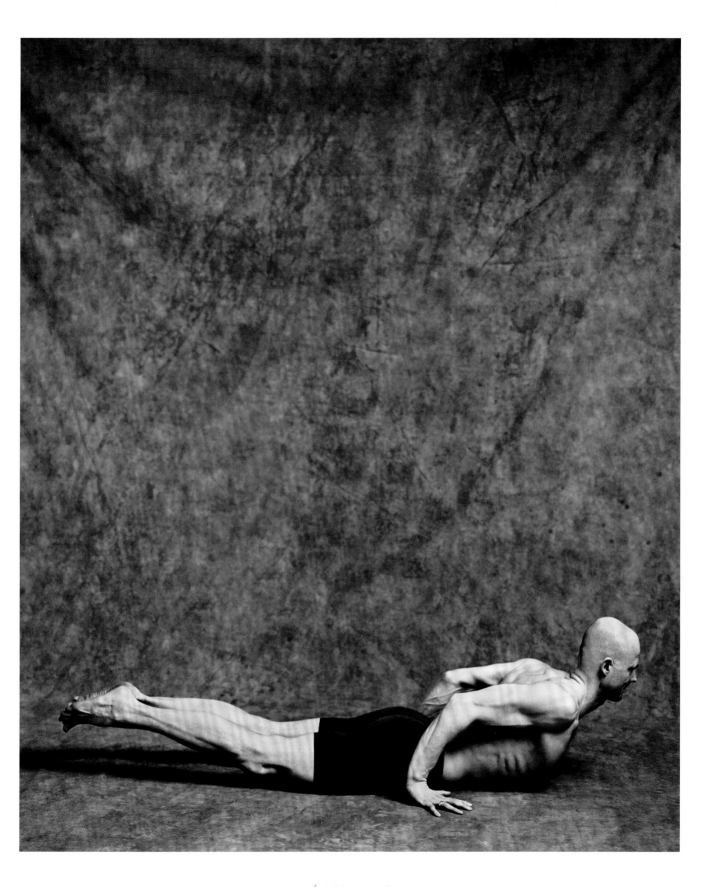

Śalabhāsana B

शलभासन २

Bhekāsana

भेकासन

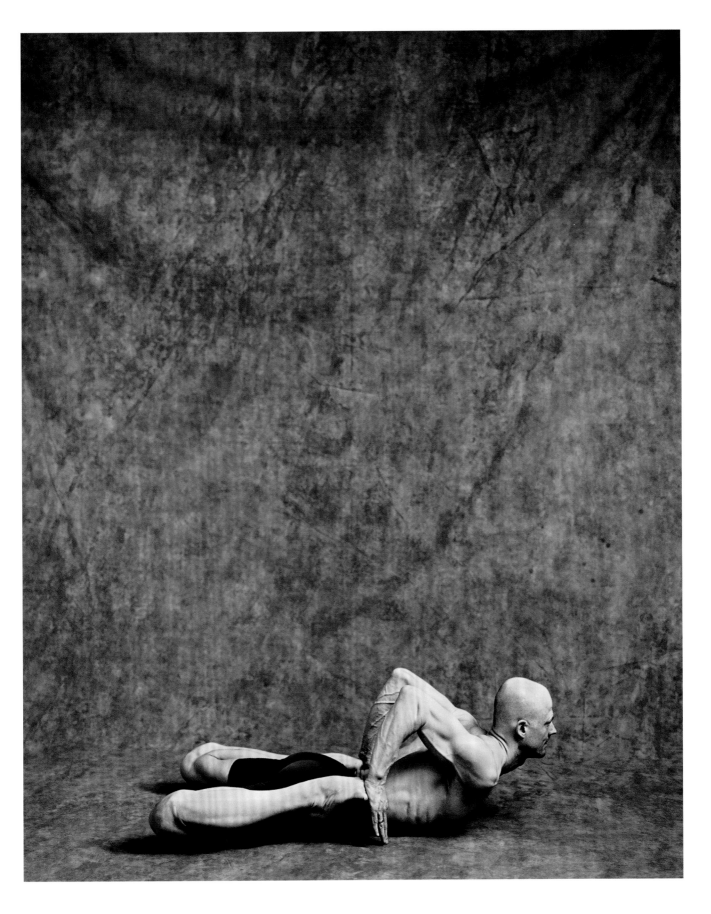

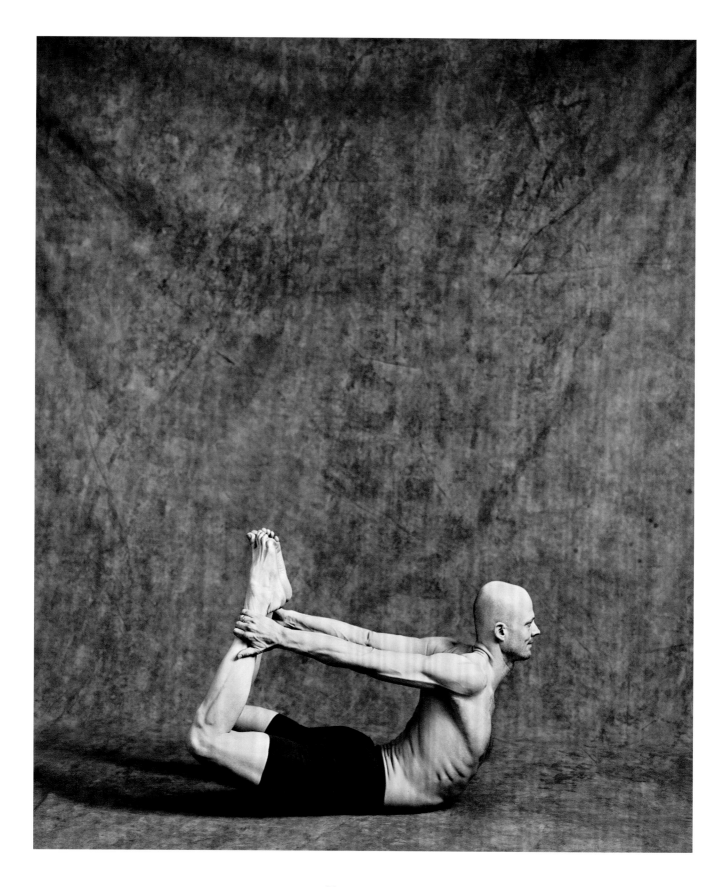

Dhanurāsana

धनुरासन

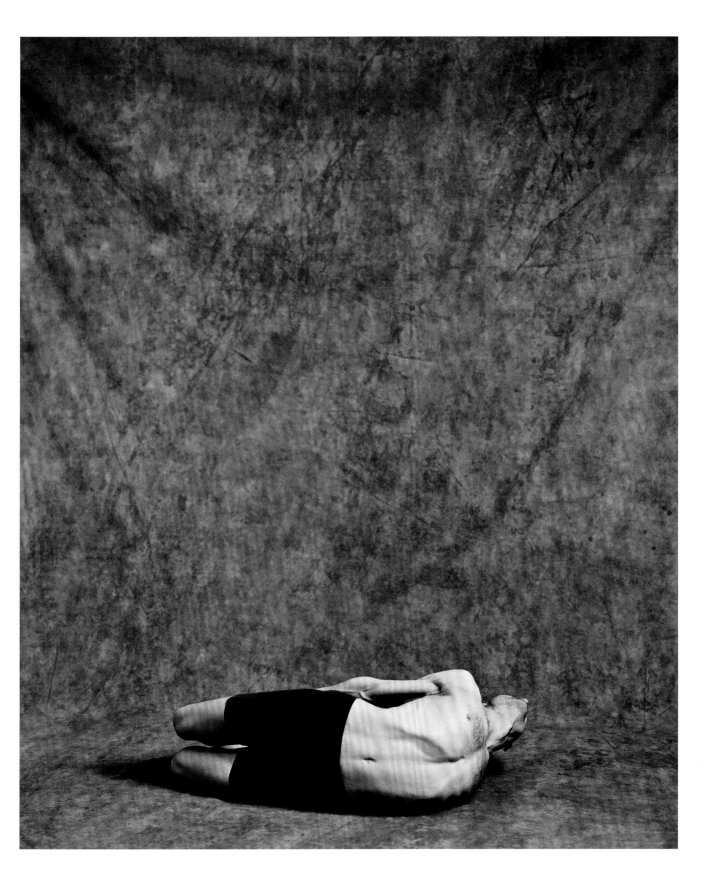

Pārśva Dhanurāsana

पार्श्वधनुरासन

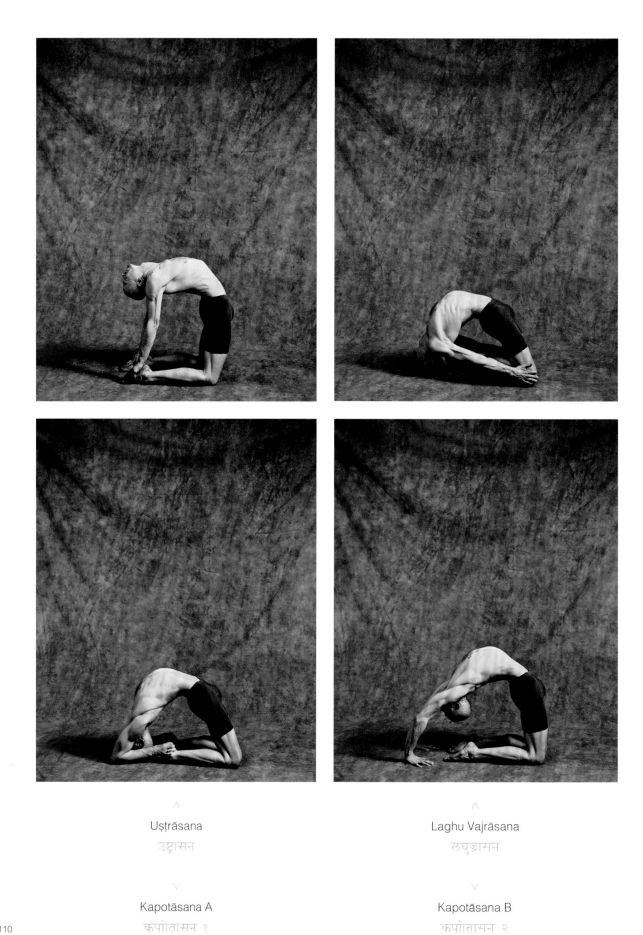

Uṣṭrāsana

उष्ट्रासन

Laghu Vajrāsana

लघुव्रज्रासन

Kapotāsana A

कपोतासन १

Kapotāsana B

कपोतासन २

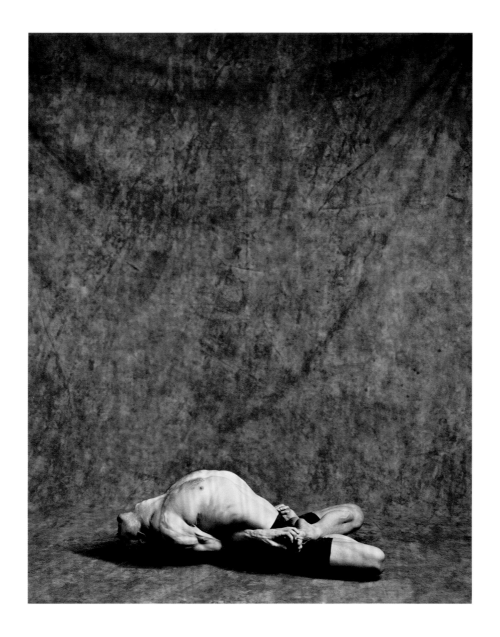

Supta Vajrāsana

सुप्तवज्रासन

Bakāsana

बकासन

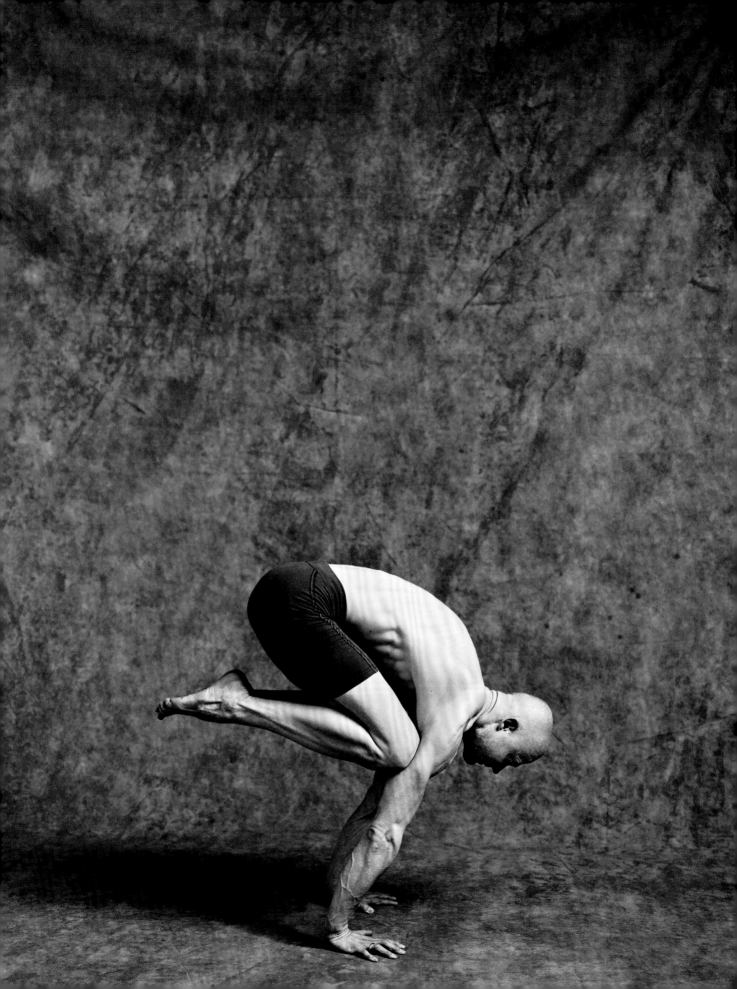

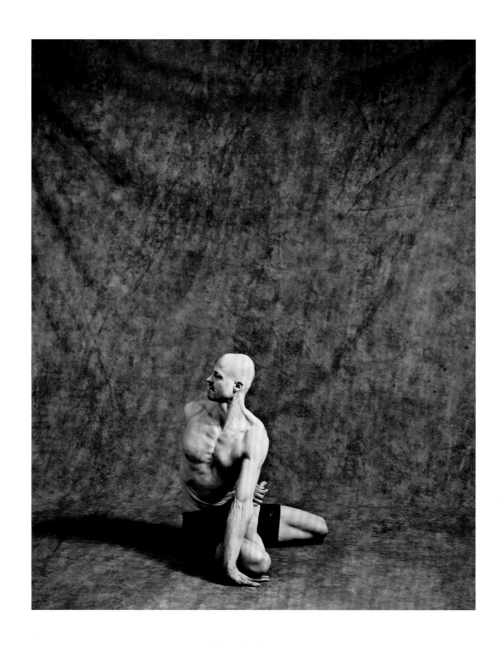

Bharadvājāsana

भरद्वाजासन

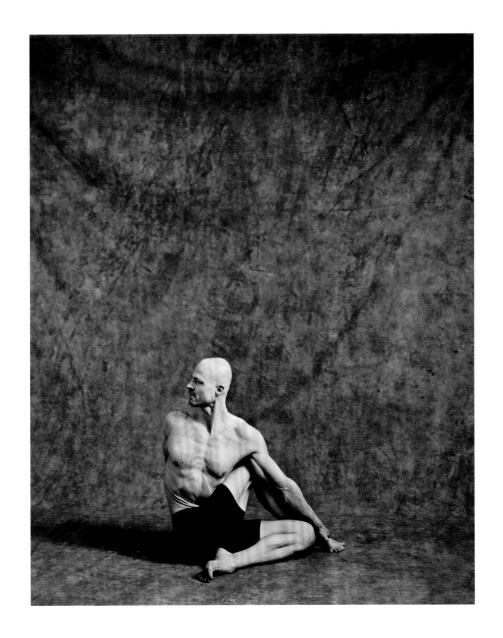

Ardha Matsyendrāsana

अधयमत्स्रोन्द्रासन

Eka Pāda Śīrṣāsana

एकपादशीर्षासन

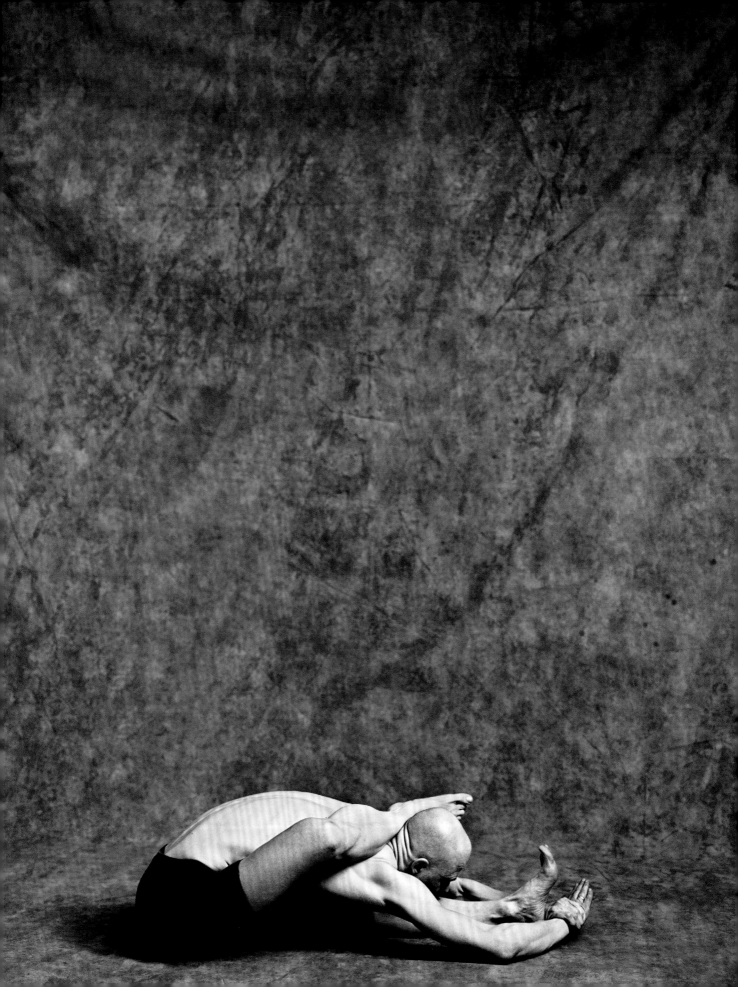

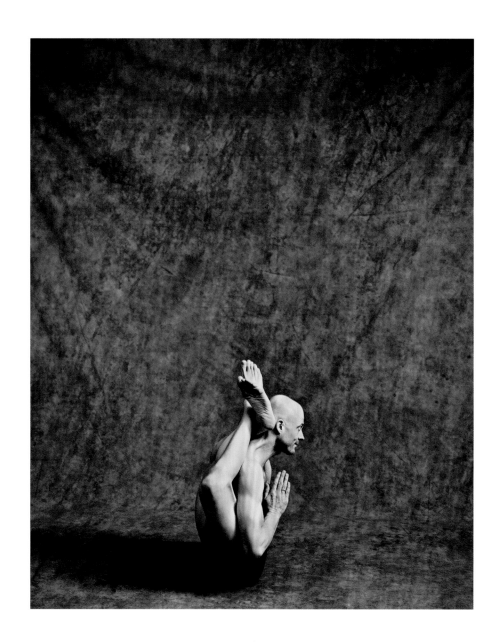

Dvi Pāda Śīrṣāsana

द्विपादशीर्षासन

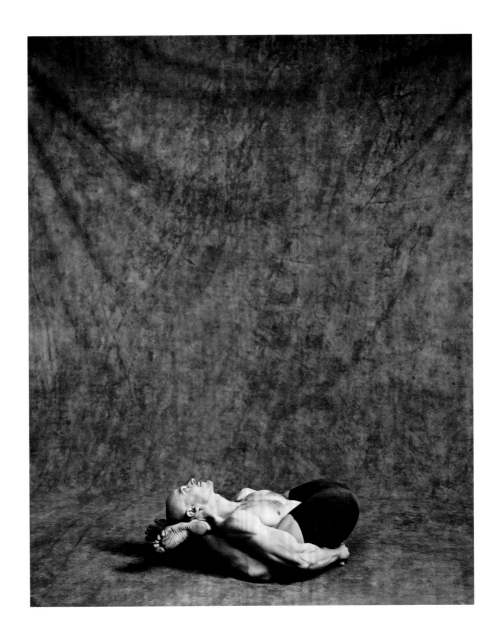

Yoga Nidrāsana

योगनिद्रासन

Tiṭṭibhāsana A

टिट्टिभासन १

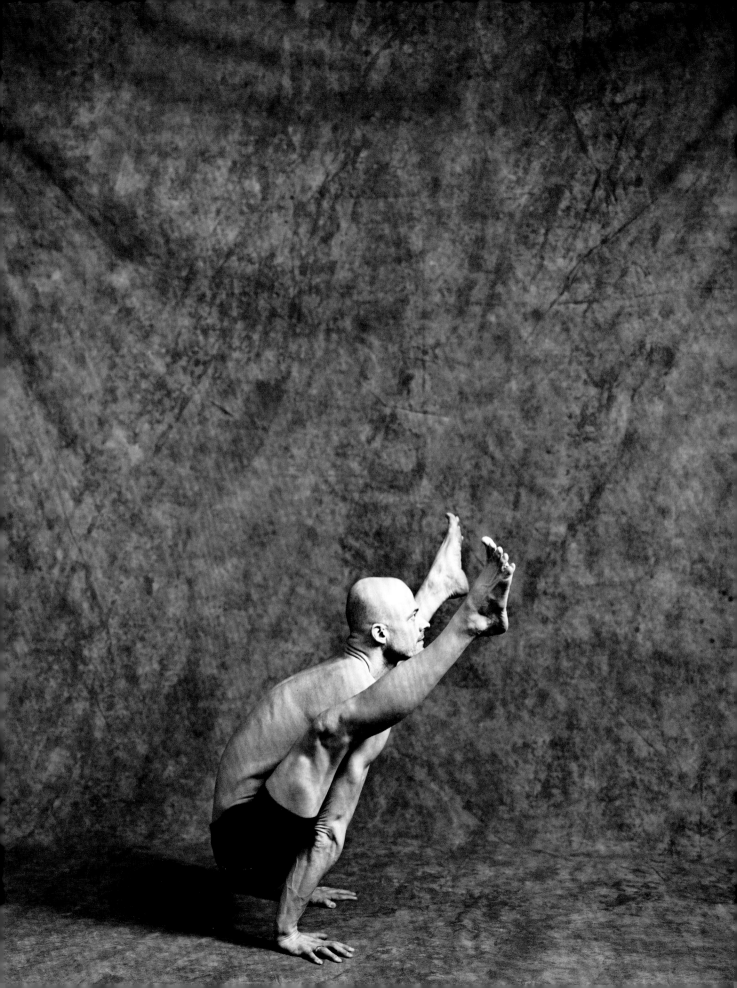

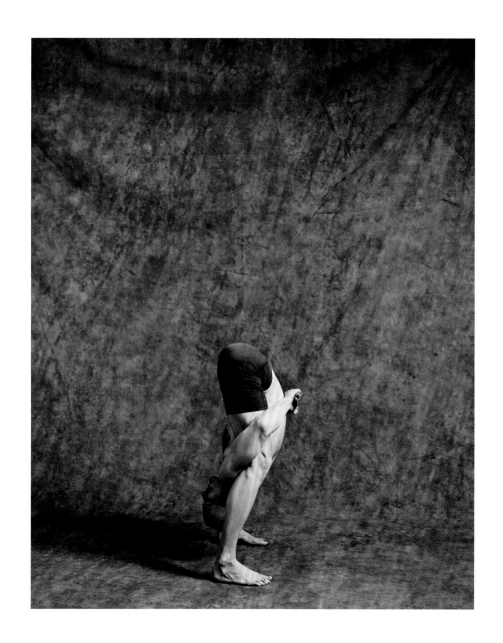

Tiṭṭibhāsana B

टिट्टिभासन २

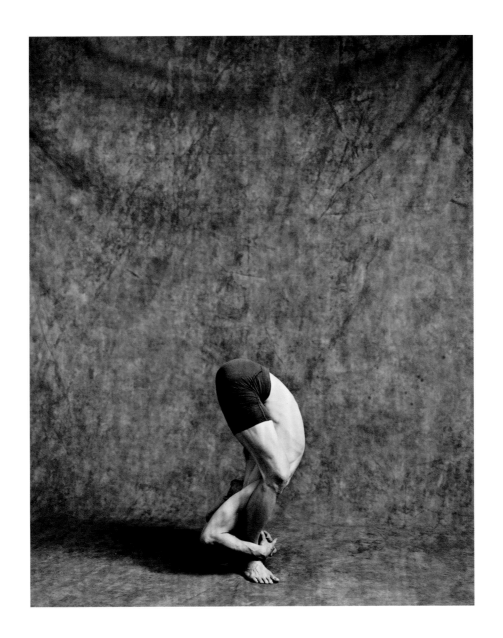

Tiṭṭibhāsana C

टिट्टिभासन ३

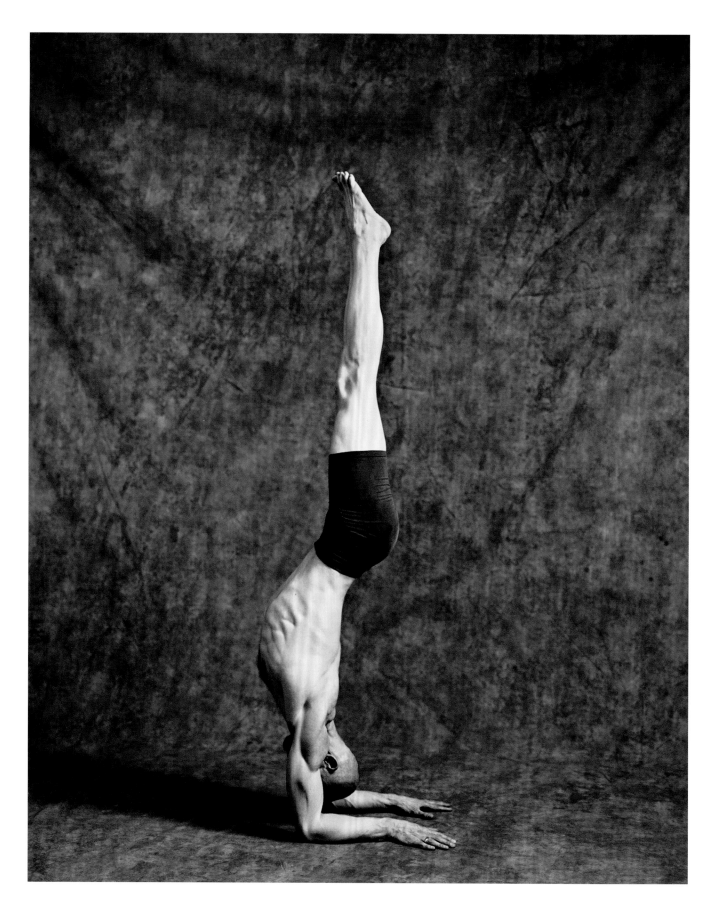

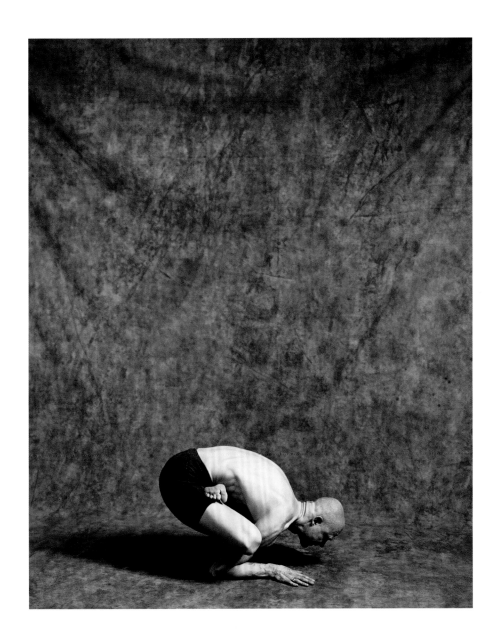

Karāndāvāsana

करन्दासन

<

Piñcha Mayūrāsana

पिञ्चमयूरासन

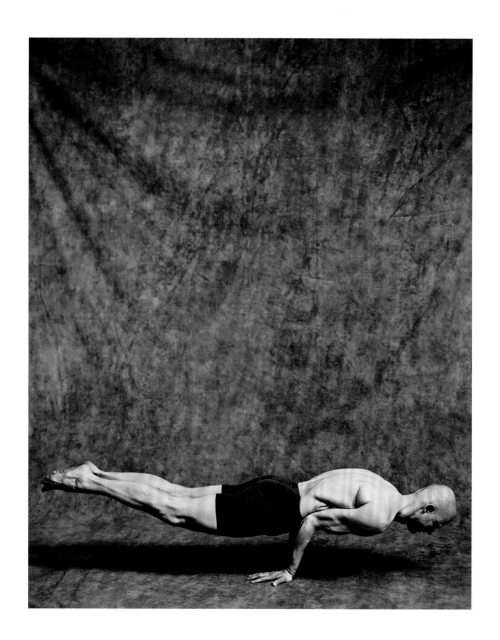

Mayūrāsana

मयूरासन

>

Nakrāsana

नक्रासन

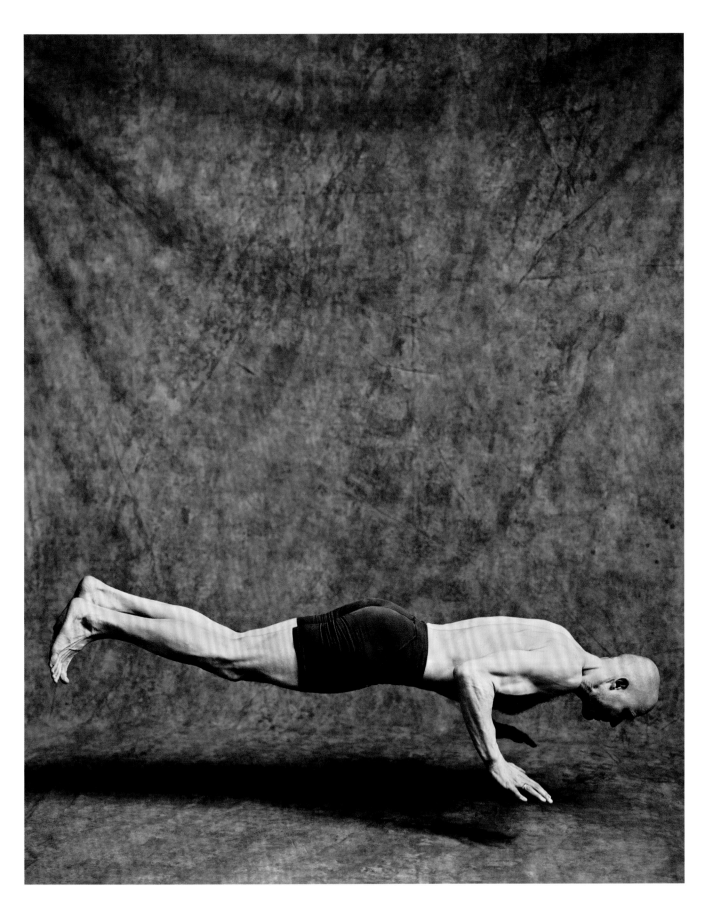

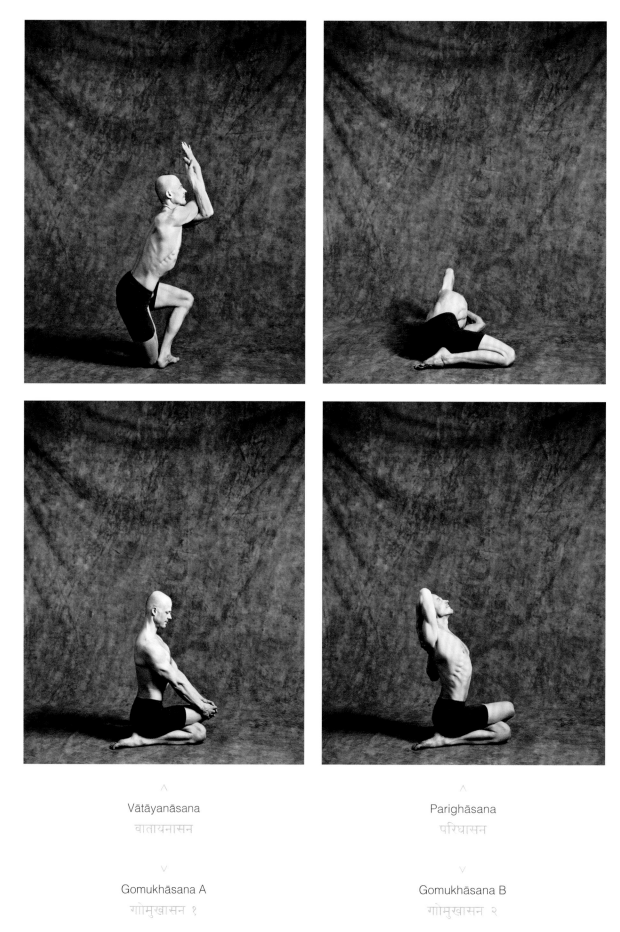

Vātāyanāsana

वातायनासन

Parighāsana

परिघासन

Gomukhāsana A

गोमुखासन १

Gomukhāsana B

गोमुखासन २

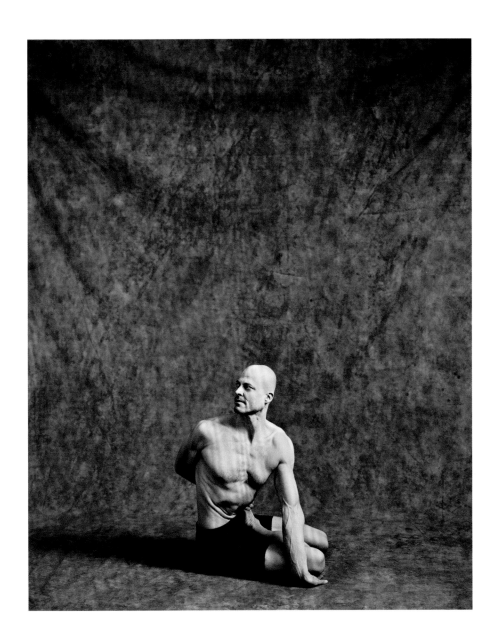

Suptordhva Pāda Vajrāsana

सुप्तोर्ध्वपादवज्रासन

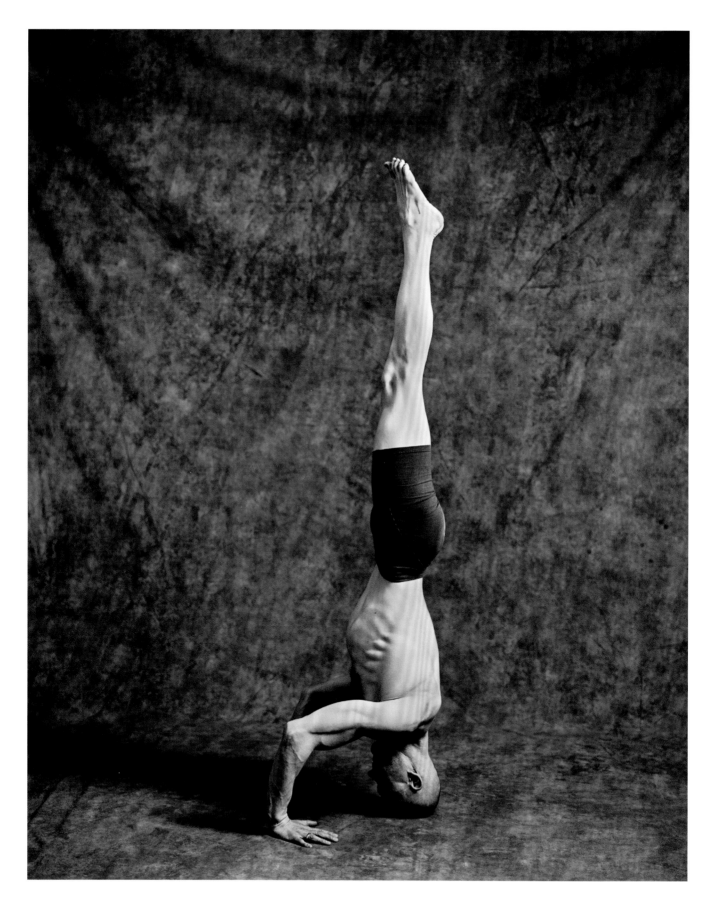

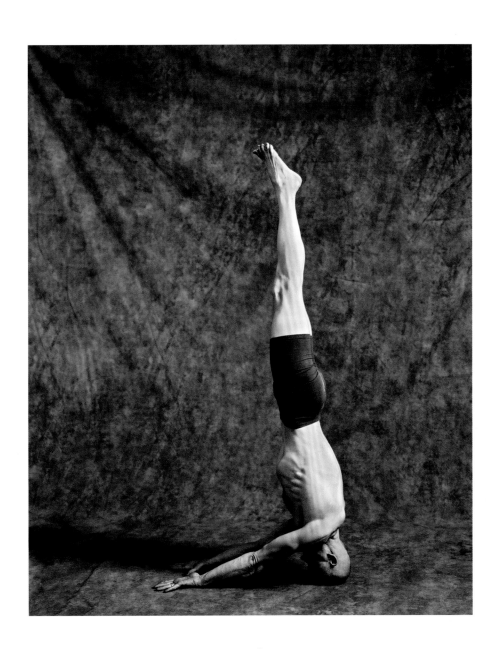

Mukta Hasta Śīrṣāsana B

मुक्तहस्तशीर्षासन २

<

Mukta Hasta Śīrṣāsana A

मुक्तहस्तशीर्षासन १

Mukta Hasta Śīrṣāsana C

मुक्तहस्तशीर्षासन ३

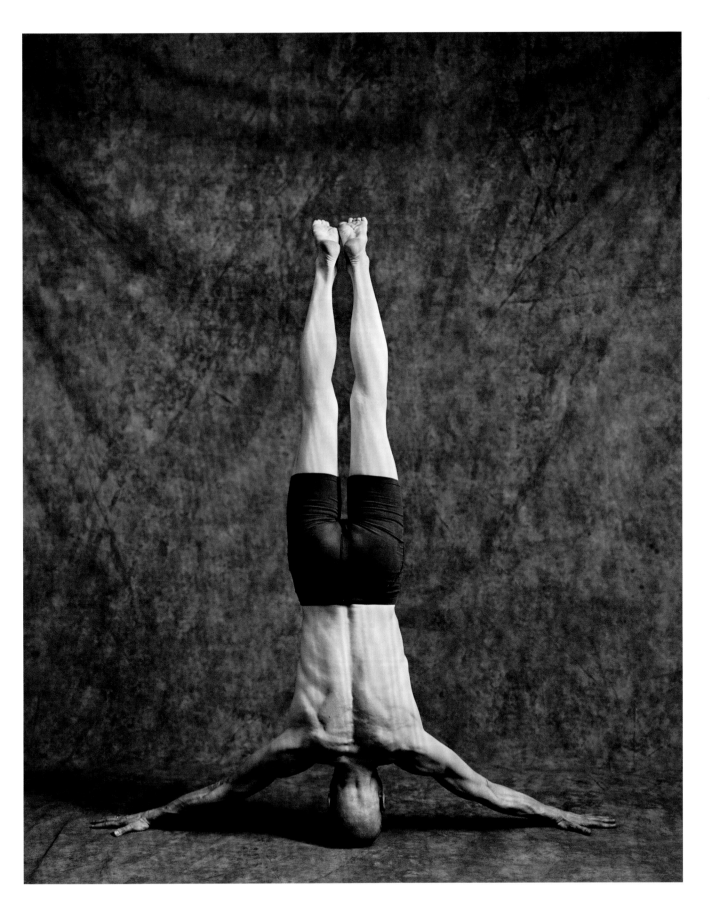

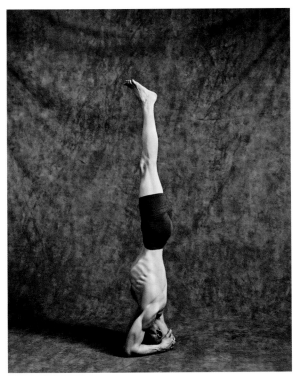

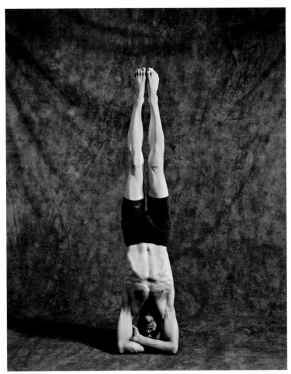

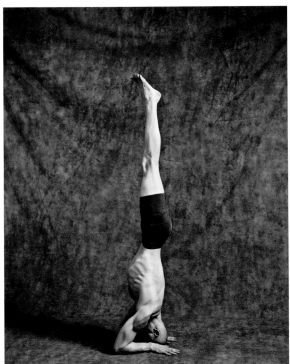

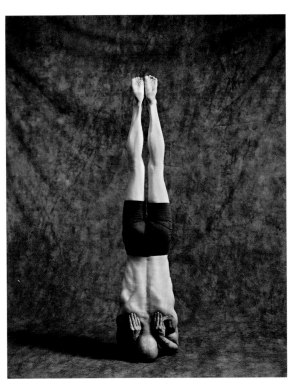

∧

Baddha Hasta Śīrṣāsana A

बद्धहस्तशीर्षासन १

∧

Baddha Hasta Śīrṣāsana B

बद्धहस्तशीर्षासन २

∨

Baddha Hasta Śīrṣāsana C

बद्धहस्तशीर्षासन ३

∨

Baddha Hasta Śīrṣāsana D

बद्धहस्तशीर्षासन ४

Ūrdhva Dhanurāsana

ऊर्ध्वधनुरासन

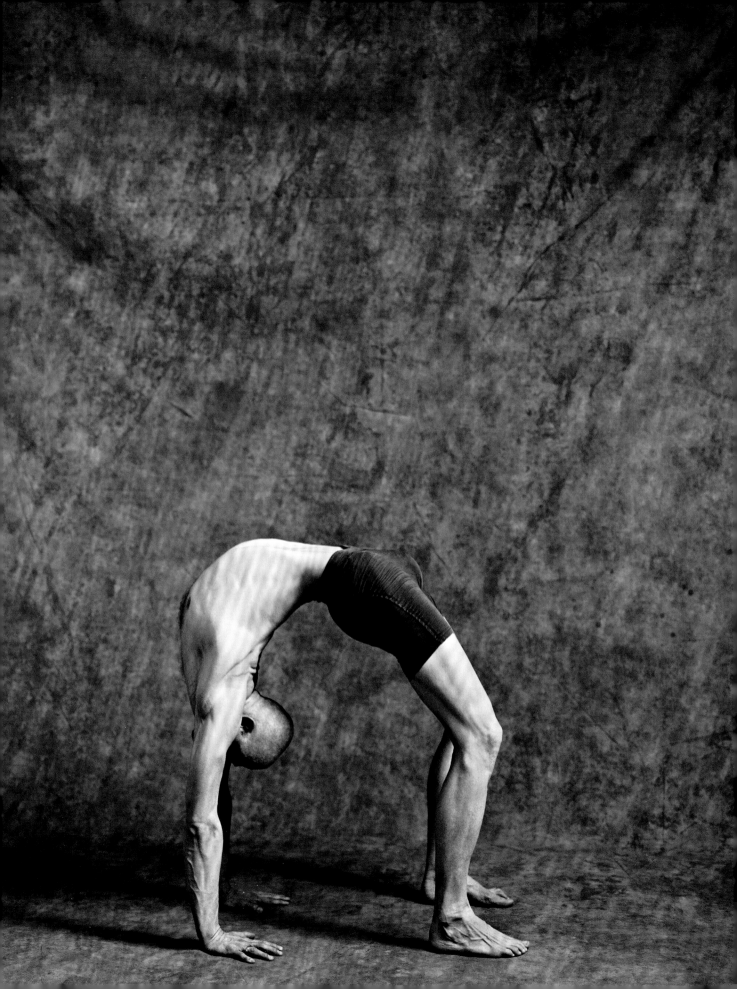

Advanced A

Sthira Bhaga A

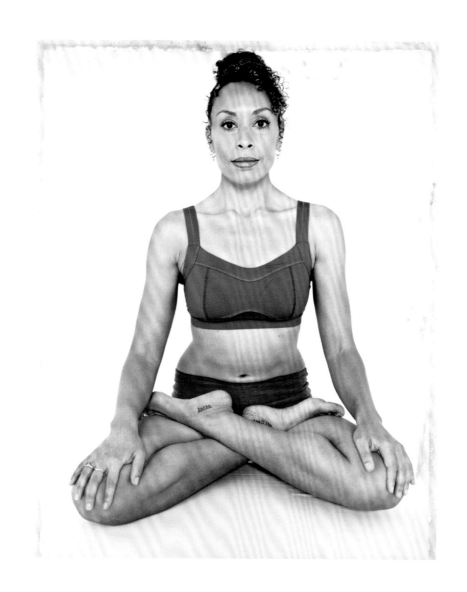

Laruga Glaser

It's the mouth

Housing the master of language

It's the heart

Where the inner voice speaks

When intuition and mind are synchronized

You learn to listen before you speak

When strong convictions push forward

You learn to stand before you walk

A good debater to clarify thoughts

An excellent counsellor to inspire advice

A convincing teacher to strengthen moves

The constant demand for challenges in life

It's a language of craft

To do the profession down to the last detail

The act of self-discipline

When the idealist meets perfectionism

It's the lips

Reflecting the powerful need for love

It's the soul

Where the playful romantic says

Forever young at heart I remain

Viśvāmitrāsana

विश्वामित्रासन

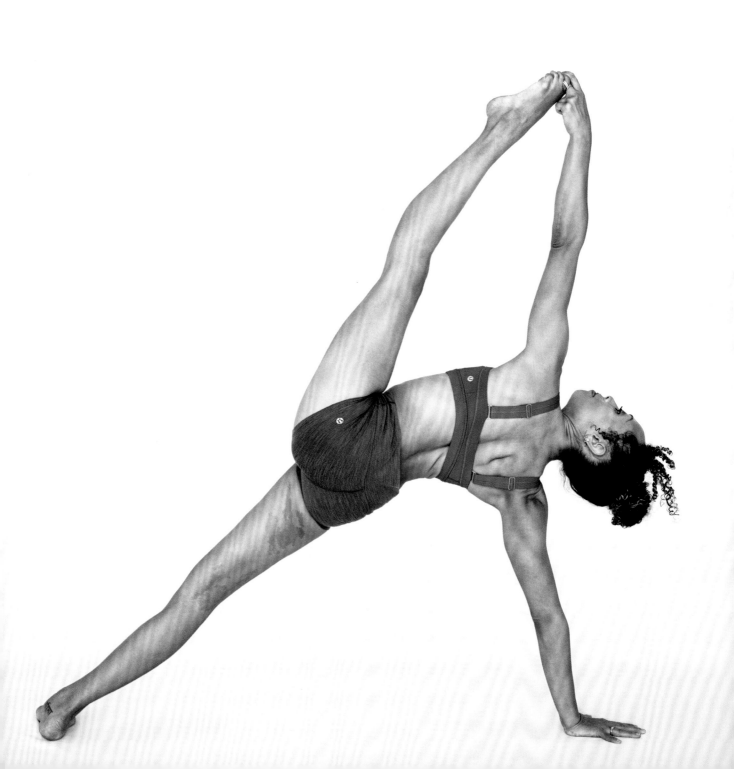

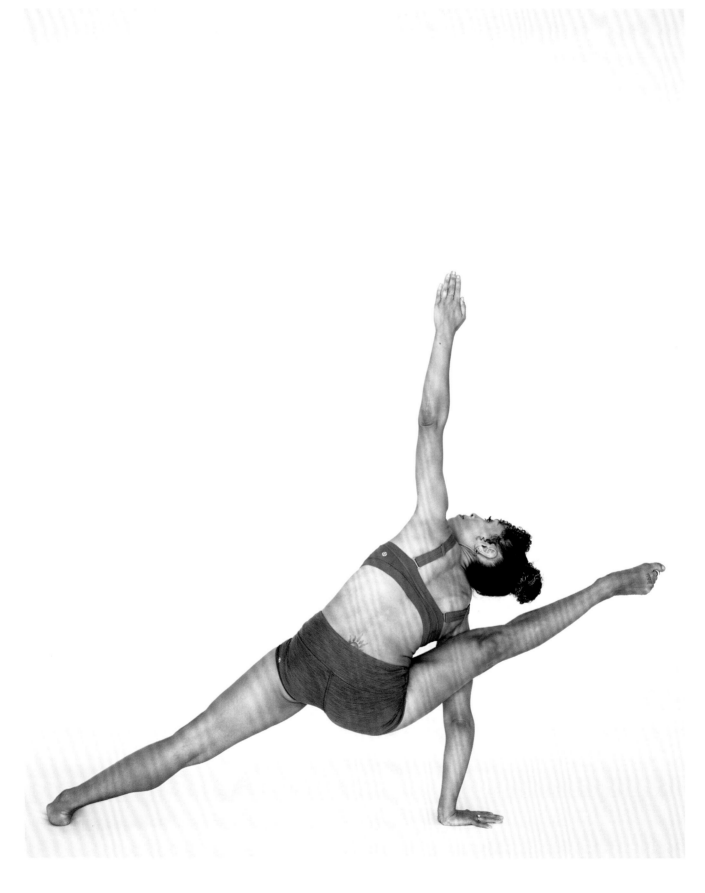

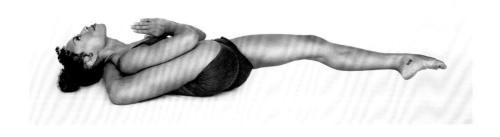

Kaśyapāsana

कश्यपासन

<

Vasiṣṭhāsana

वसिष्ठासन

Cakorāsana

चकोरासन

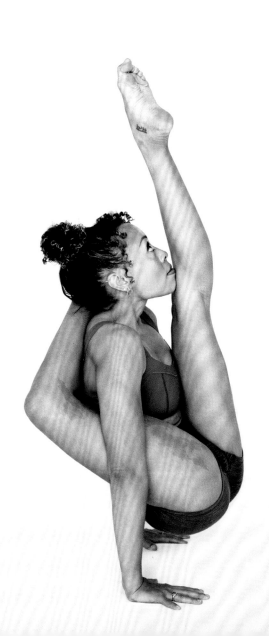

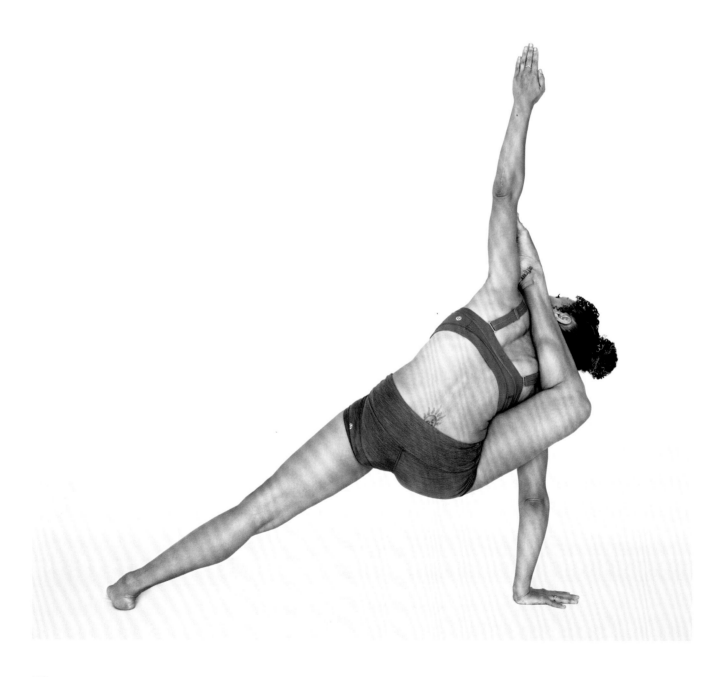

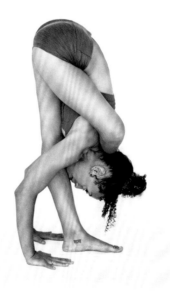

Skandāsana

स्कन्दासन

<

Bhairavāsana

भैरवासन

Durvāsana

दर्वासन

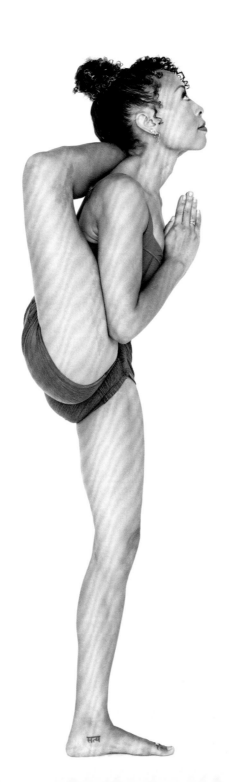

Ūrdhva Kukkuṭāsana

ऊर्ध्वकुक्कुटासन

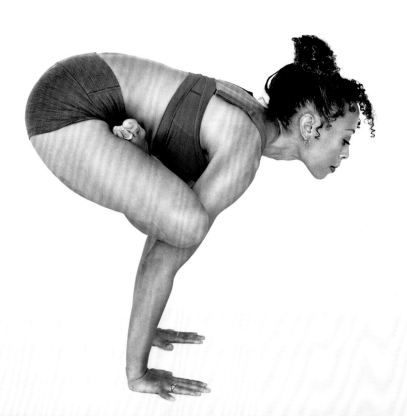

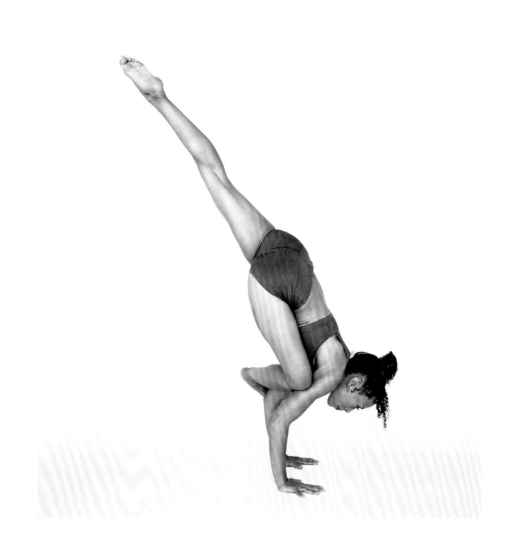

Gālavāsana

गालवासन

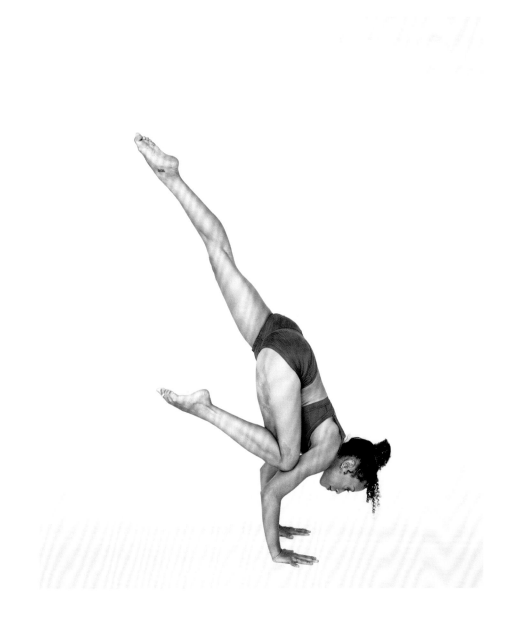

Eka Pāda Bakāsana A

एकपादबकासन १

Eka Pāda Bakāsana B

एकपादबकासन २

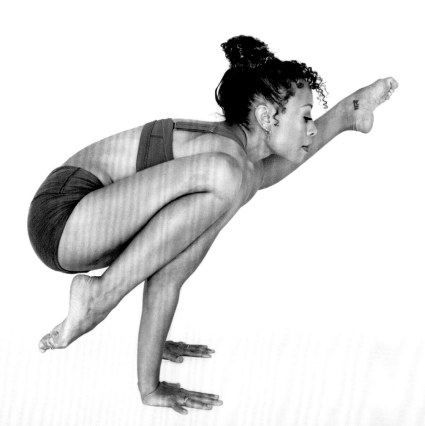

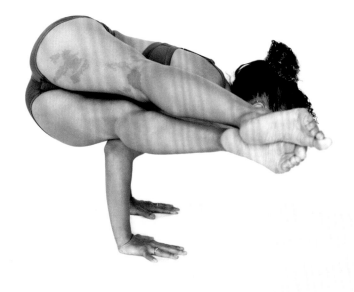

Kauṇḍinyāsana A

कौण्डिन्यासन १

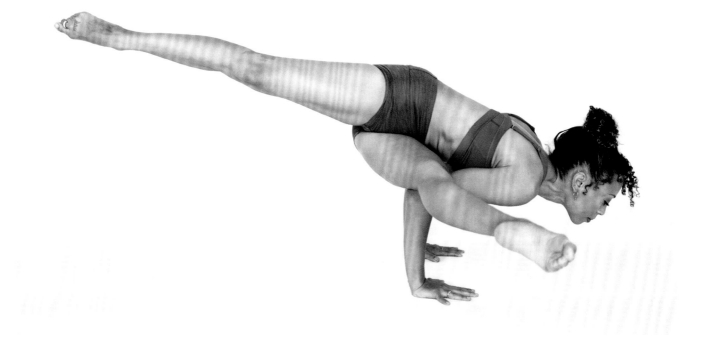

Kauṇḍinyāsana B

कोण्डिन्यासन २

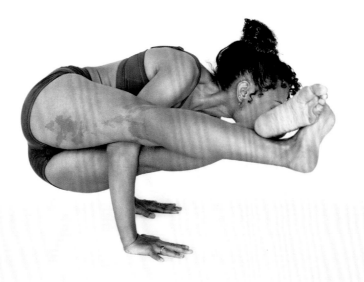

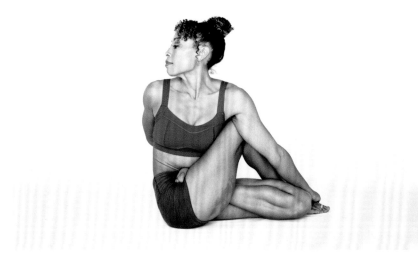

Pūrṇa Matsyendrāsana

पूर्णमत्स्येन्द्रासन

<

Aṣṭāvakrāsana

अष्टवक्रासन

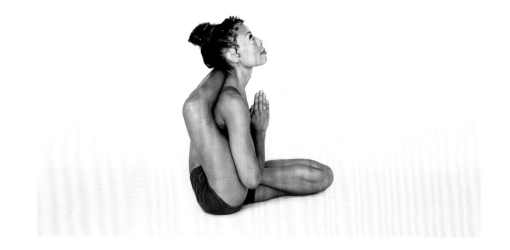

Virañcyāsana A

विरञ्च्यासन १

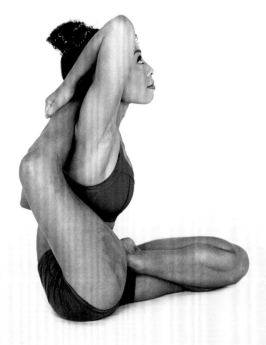

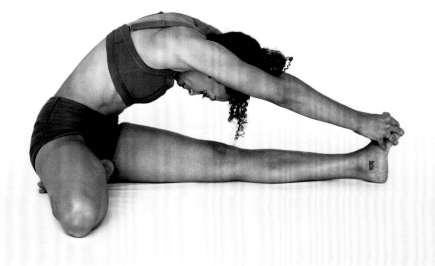

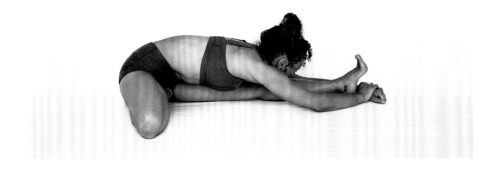

‹ ∧

Virañcyāsana B

विरञ्च्यासन २

Virañcyāsana B

विरञ्चासन २

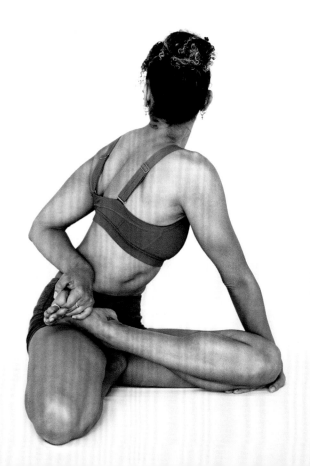

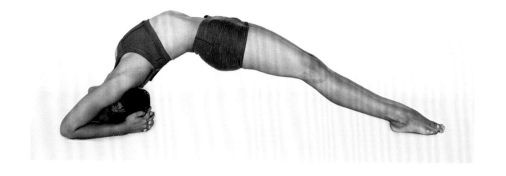

Dvi Pāda Viparīta Daṇḍāsana

द्विपादविपरीतदण्डासन

>

Eka Pāda Viparīta Daṇḍāsana

एकपादविपरीतदण्डासन

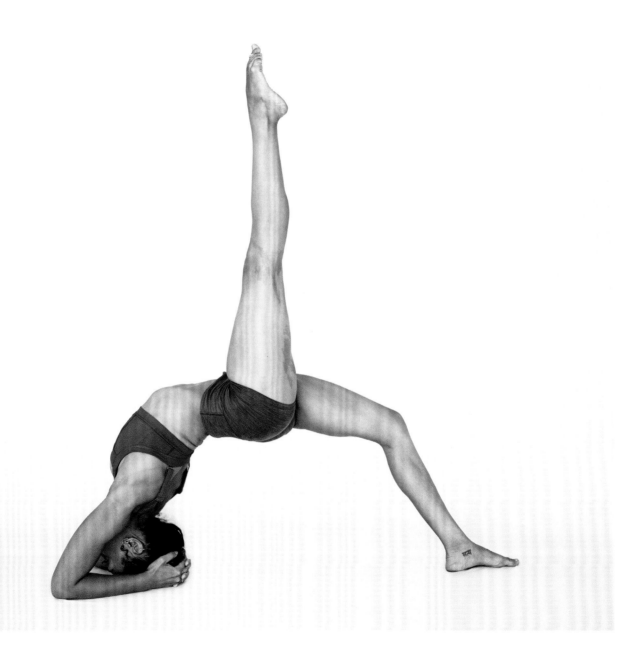

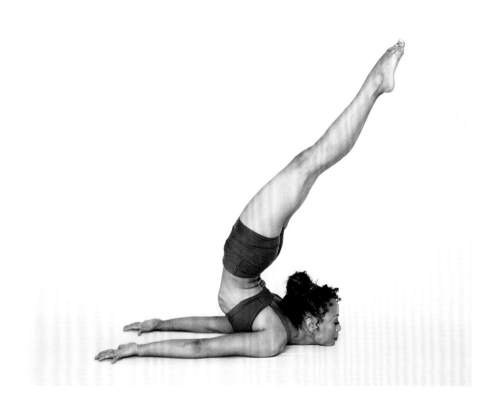

Viparīta Śalabhāsana

विपरीतशलभासन

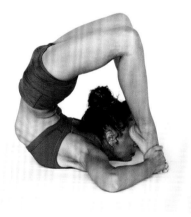

Gaṇḍa Bheruṇḍāsana

गण्डभेरुण्डासन

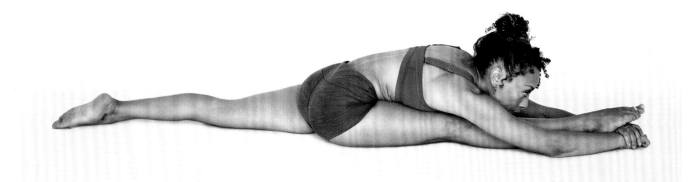

Hanumanāsana

हनुमानासन

Supta Trivikramāsana

सुप्तत्रिविक्रमासन

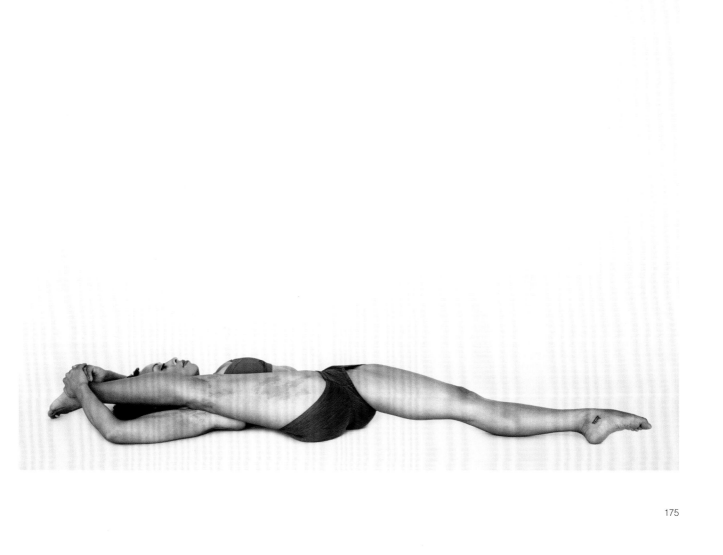

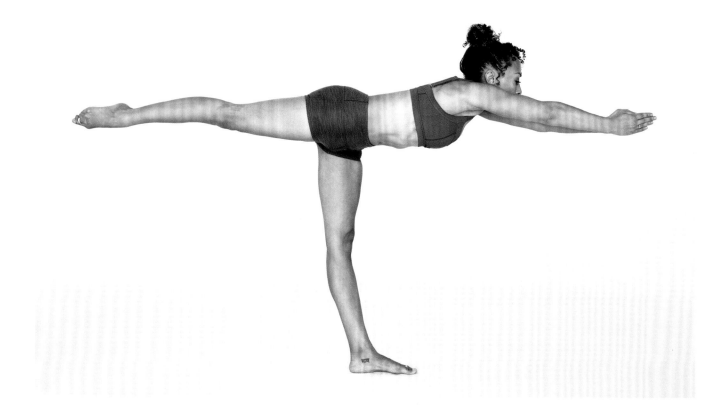

Digāsana A

दिगासन १

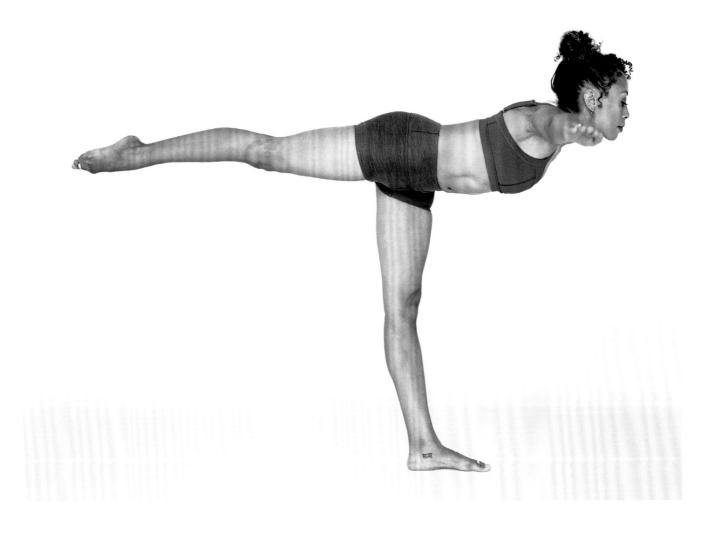

Digāsana B

दिगासन २

Utthita Trivikramāsana

उत्थितत्रिविक्रमासन

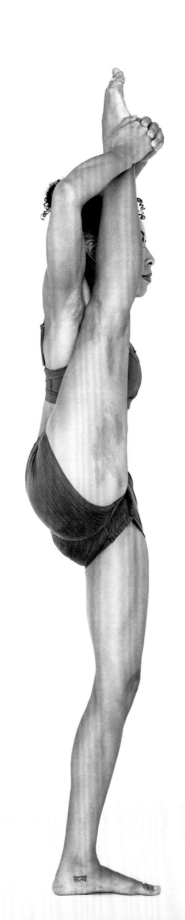

Naṭa Rājāsana

नटराजासन

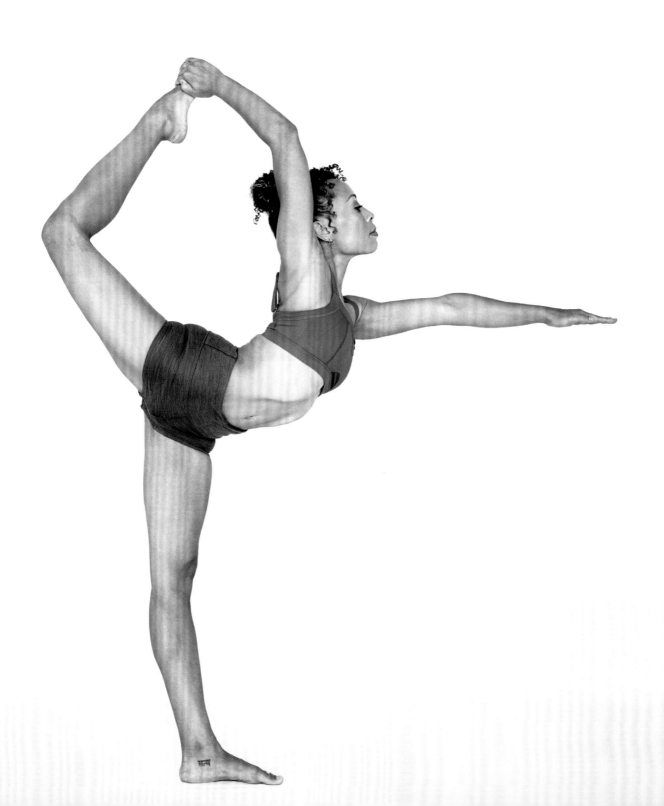

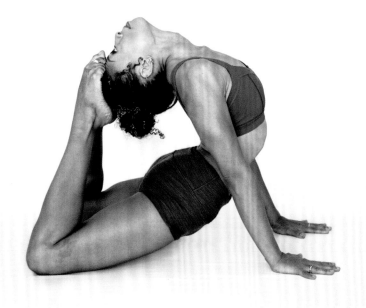

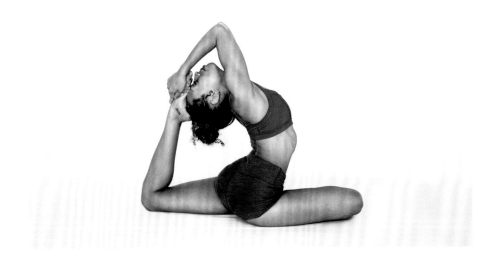

Eka Pāda Rāja Kapotāsana

एकपादराजकपोतासन

<

Rāja Kapotāsana

राजकपोतासन

Ūrdhva Dhanurāsana

ऊर्ध्वधनुरासन

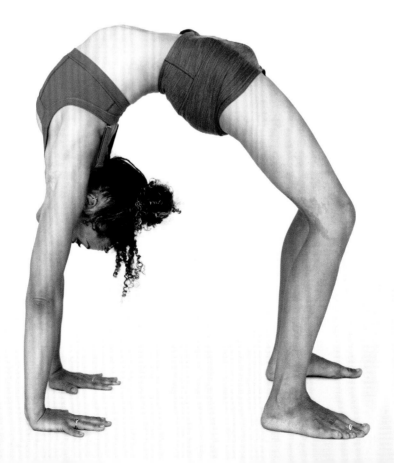

एकावन

Advanced B

Sthira Bhaga B

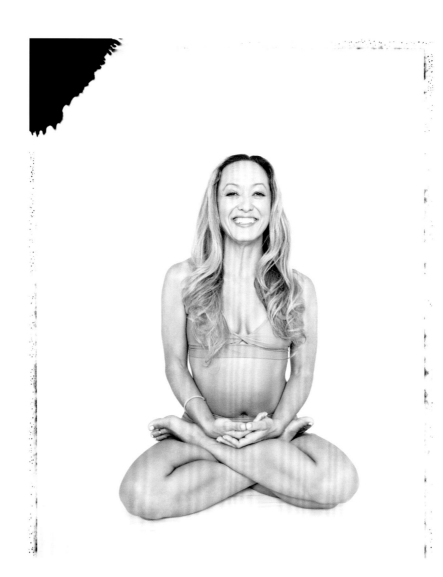

Kino MacGregor

It's honesty I adore
It's clarity I prefer
Enlightenment I strive for

The great actor
Love is communication
Words so highly valued

The fearless warrior
Let action speak for me
Obstacles are invitations

The critical thinker
Remain objective
With good reasoning power

The intuitive idealist
Need for creative expression
Desire to establish true identity

The private person
With discipline and self-control
In solitude earning self-respect

Truth leads to freedom
Freedom gives authority
Truth is God

Mūla Bandhāsana

मूलबन्धासन

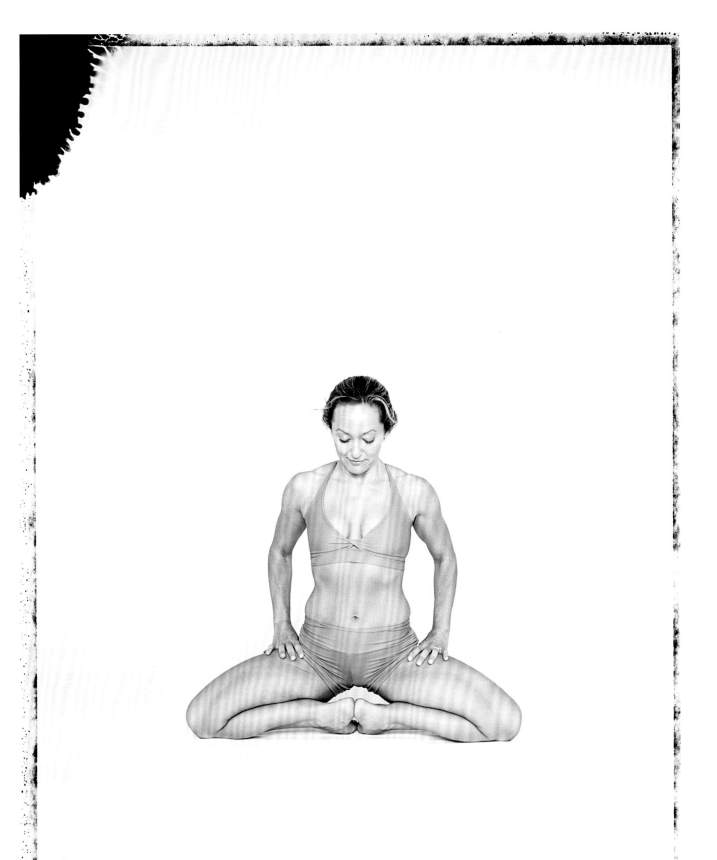

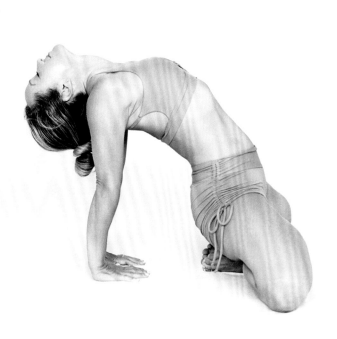

Nahuṣāsana A

नुरासन १

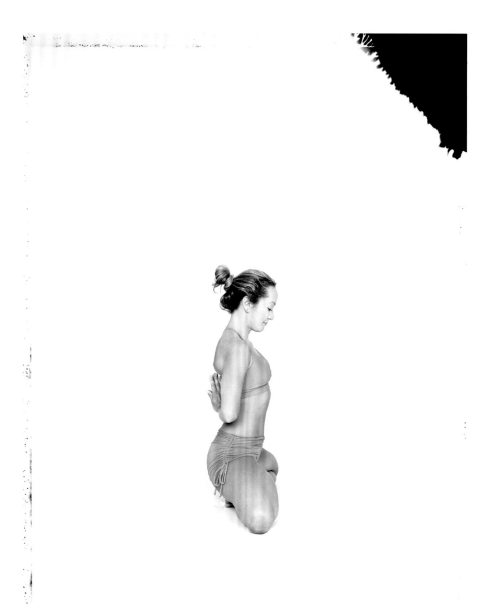

Nahuṣāsana B

नुरासन २

>

Nahuṣāsana C

नुरासन २

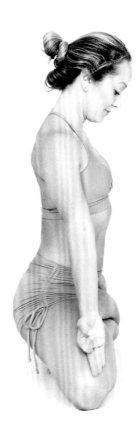

Vṛścikāsana

वृश्चिकासन

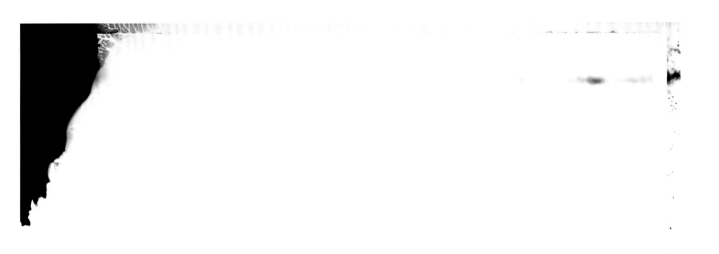

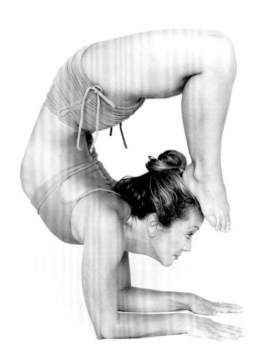

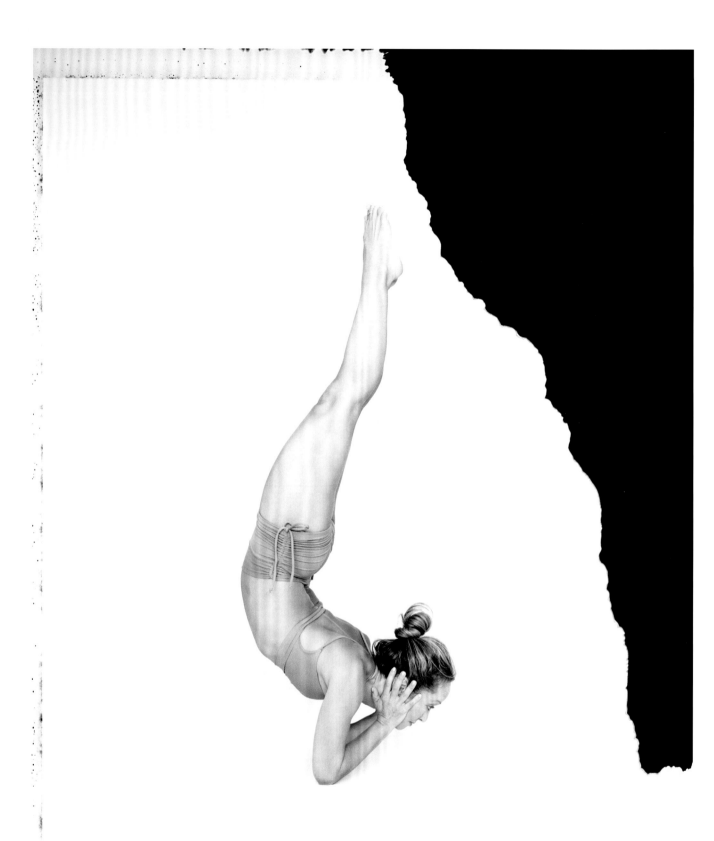

Śayanāsana

शयनासन

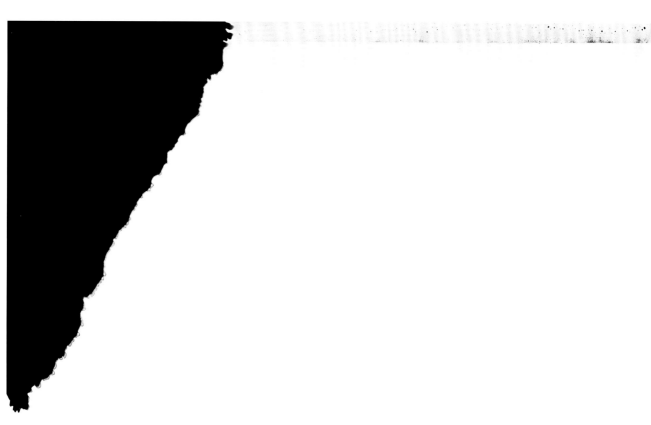

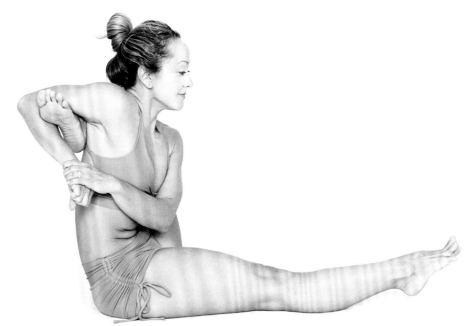

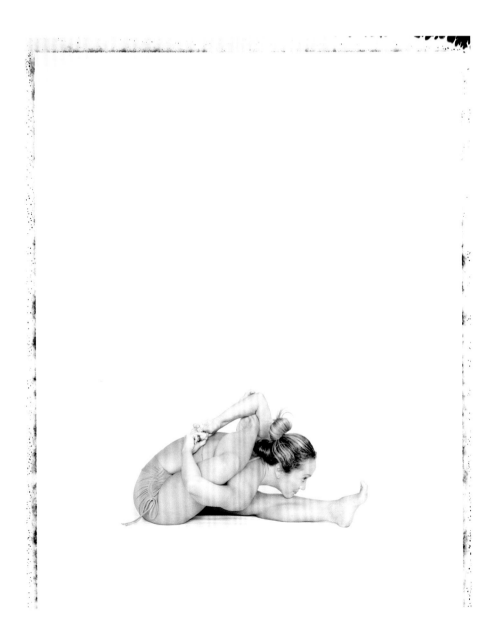

Kapilāsana

कपिलासन

Buddhāsana

बुद्धासन

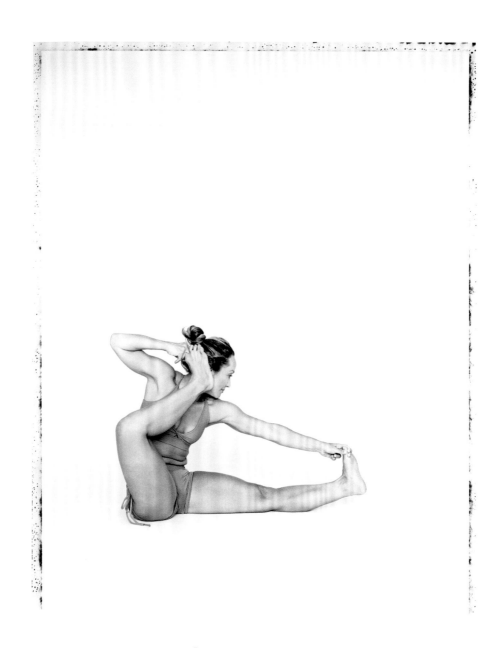

Ākarṇa Dhanurāsana A

आकर्णधनुरासन १

>

Ākarṇa Dhanurāsana B

आकर्णधनुरासन २

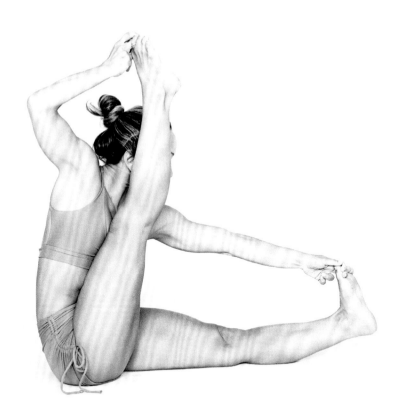

Pādāṅguṣṭha Dhanurāsana A

पादाङ्गुष्ठधनुरासन १

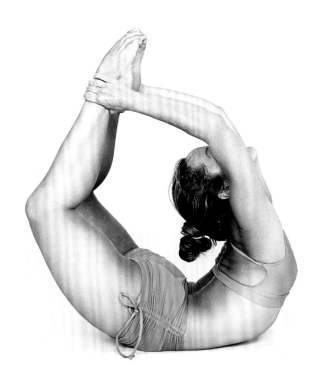

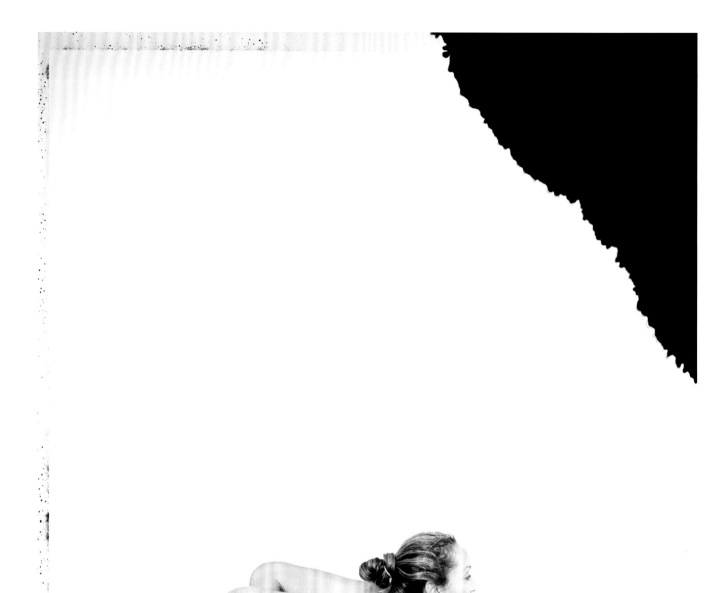

Pādāṅguṣṭha Dhanurāsana B

पादाङ्गुष्ठधनुरासन २

Marīcyāsana E

मरीच्यासन ५

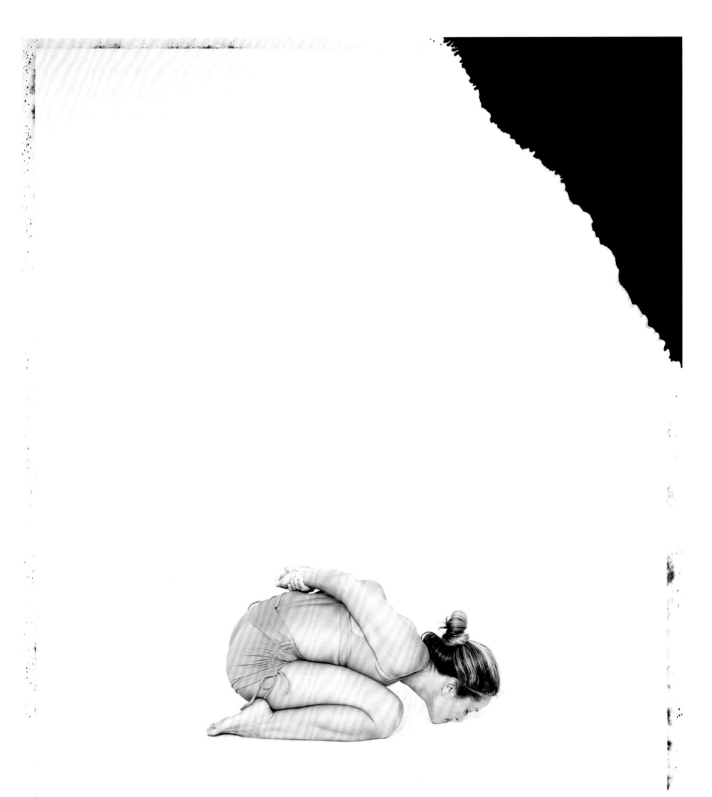

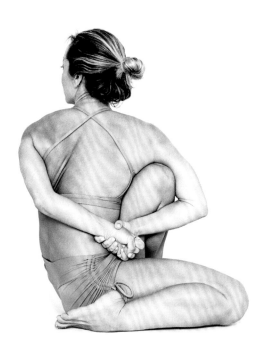

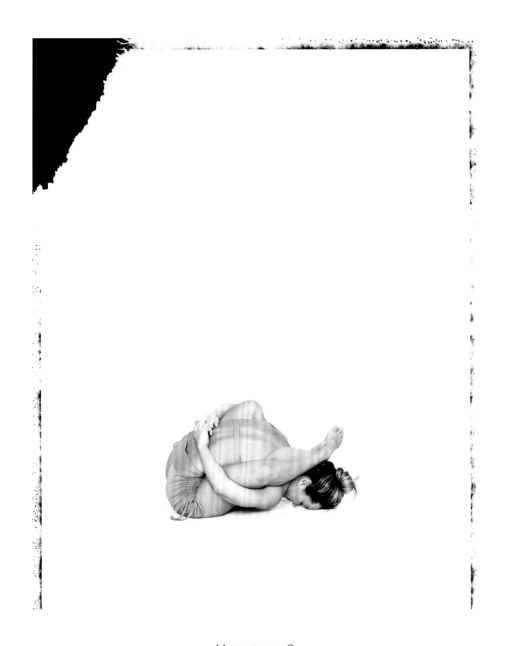

Marīcyāsana G

मरीच्यासन ७

<

Marīcyāsana F

मरीच्यासन ६

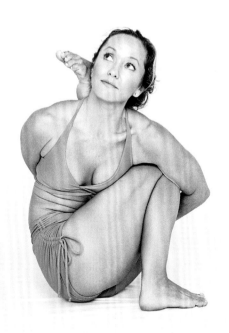

Marīcyāsana H

मरीच्यासन ८

Tāḍāsana

ताडासन

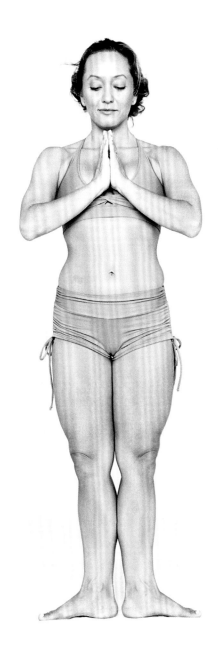

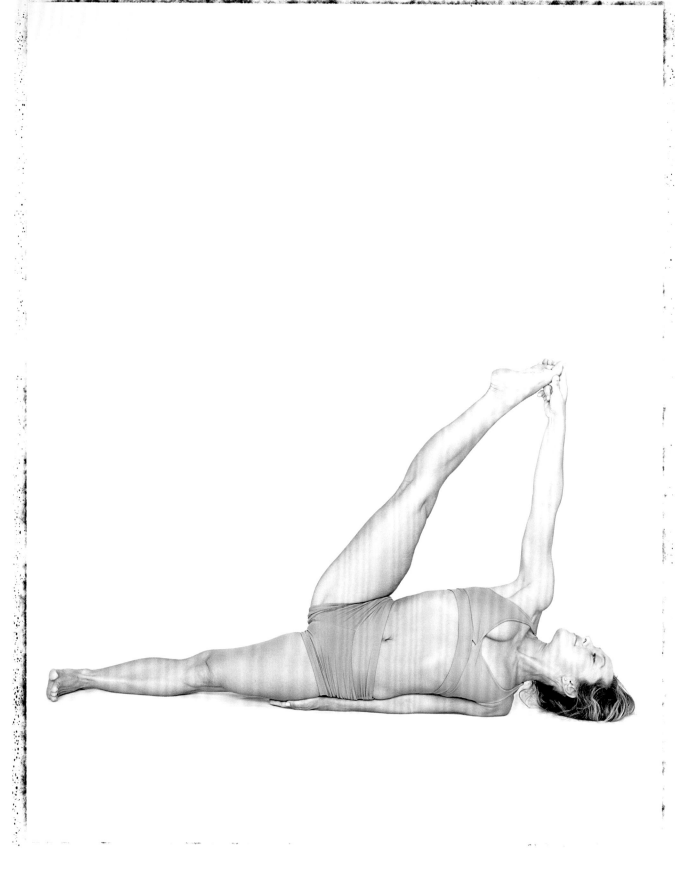

Samānāsana

समानासन

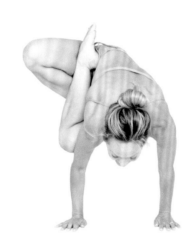

Puṇga Kukkuṭāsana

पुण्गकुक्कुटासन

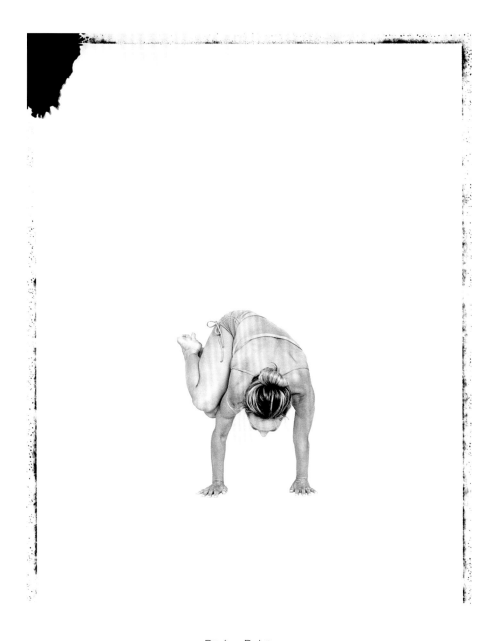

Pārśva Bakāsana

पार्श्वबकासन

Eka Pāda Dhanurāsana A

एकपादधनुरासन १

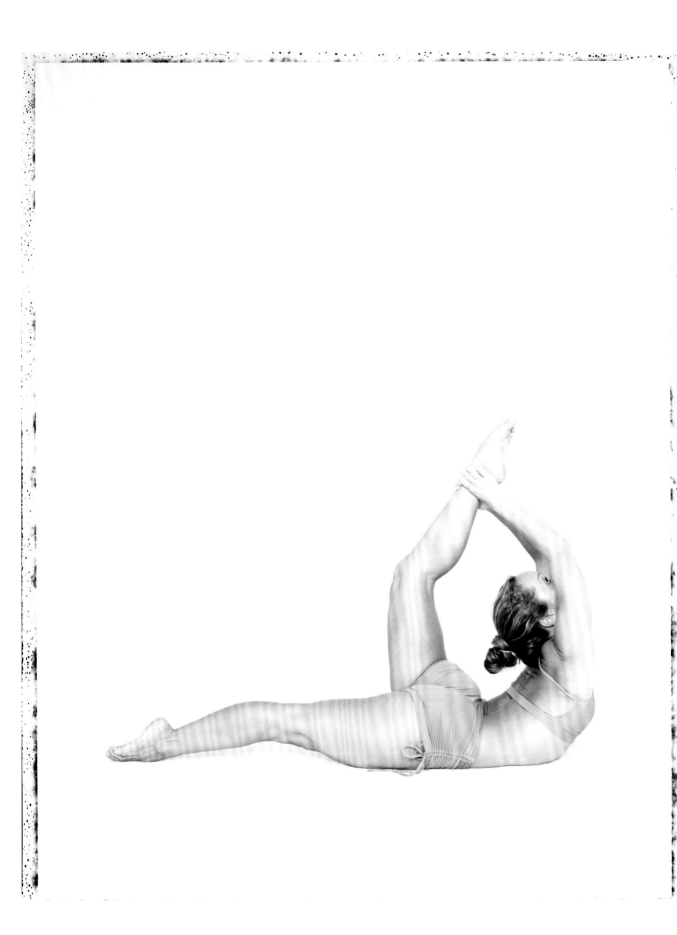

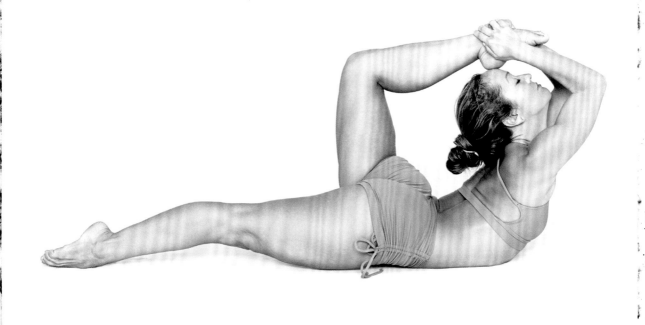

Eka Pāda Dhanurāsana B

एकपादधनुरासन २

Eka Pāda Kapotāsana A

एकपादकपोतासन १

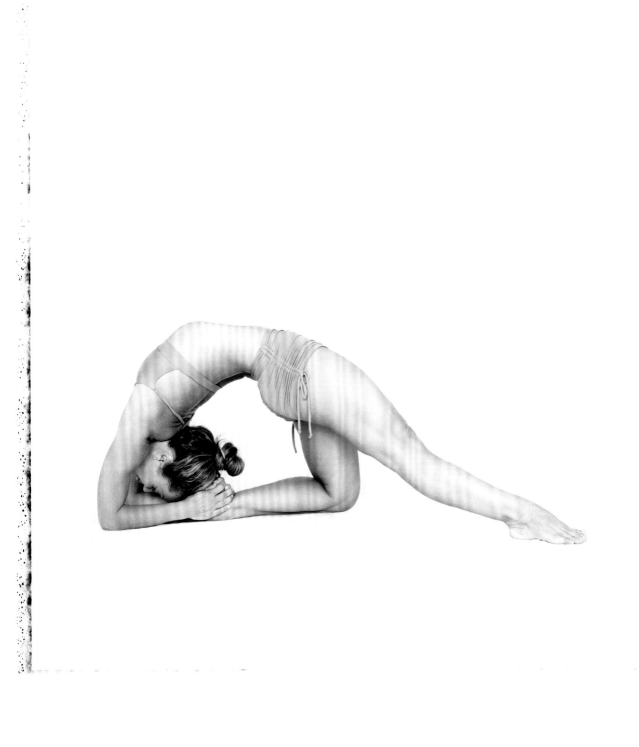

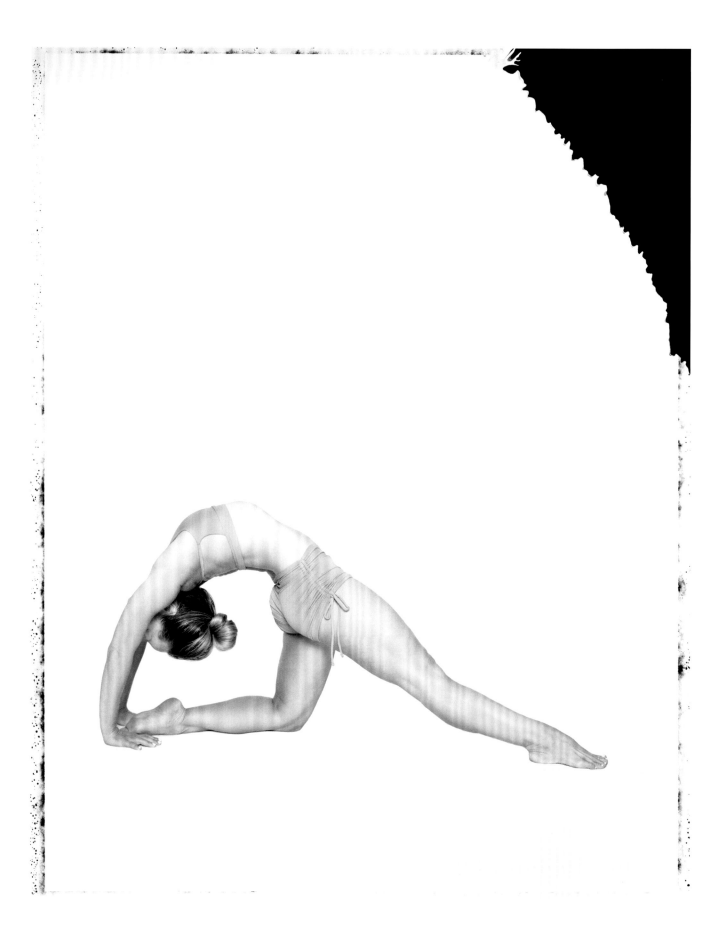

Eka Pāda Kapotāsana B

एकपादकपोतासन २

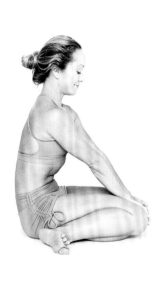

Paryaṅgāsana A

पर्यङ्कासन १

>

Paryaṅgāsana B

पर्यङ्कासन २

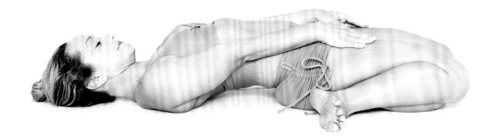

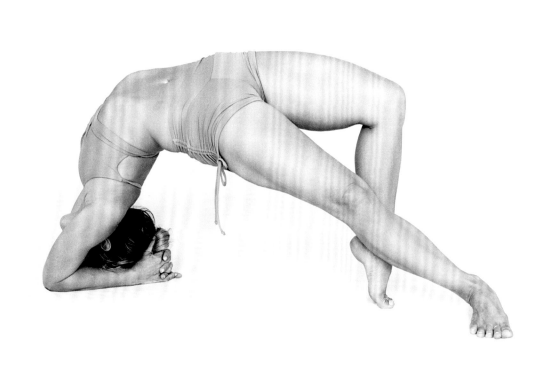

Parivṛttāsana A

परिवृत्तासन १

Parivṛttāsana B

परिवृत्तासन २

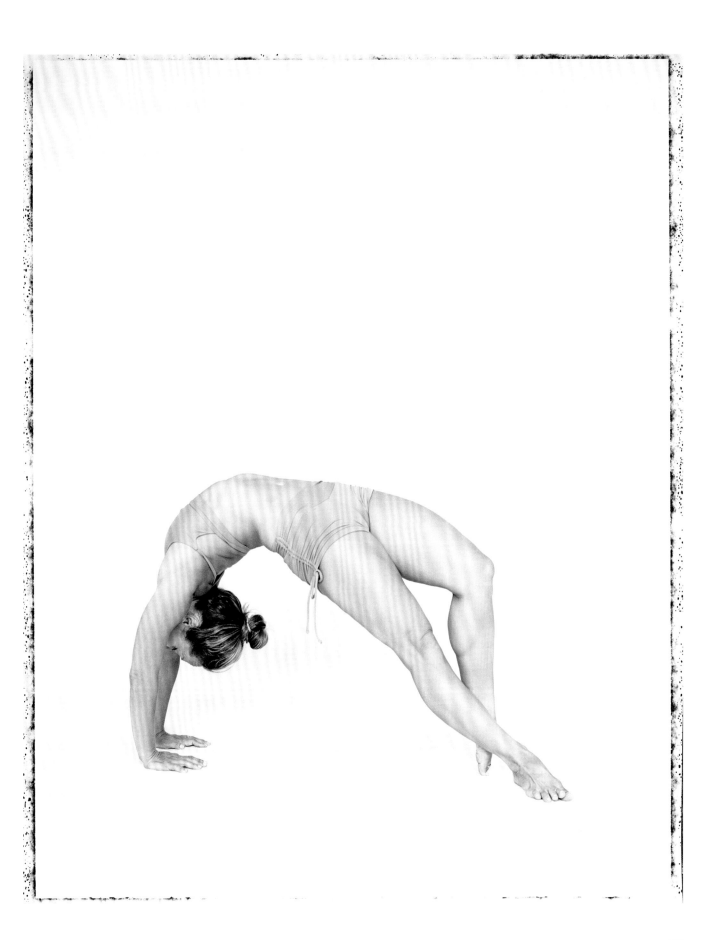

Yoni Daṇḍāsana A

योनिदण्डासन १

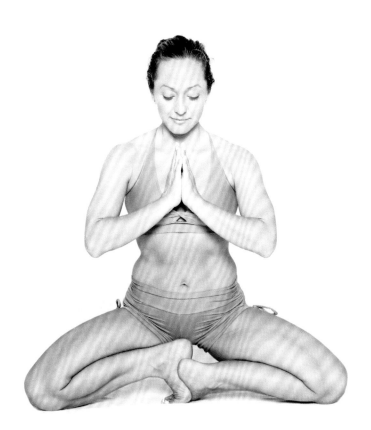

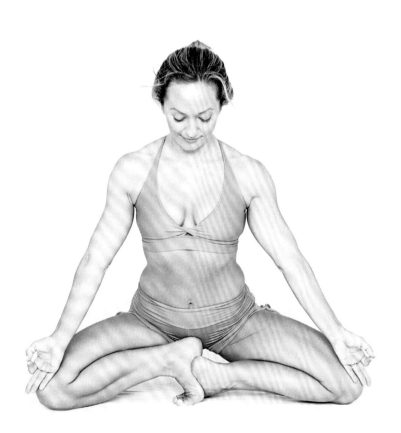

Yoni Daṇḍāsana B

योनिदण्डासन २

Yoga Daṇḍāsana

योगदण्डासन

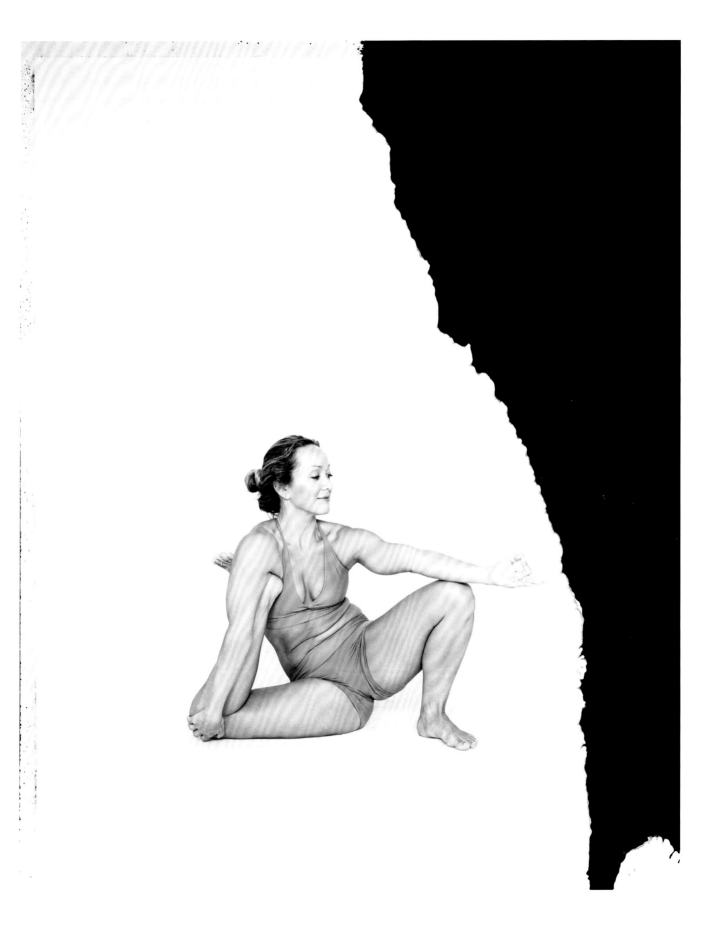

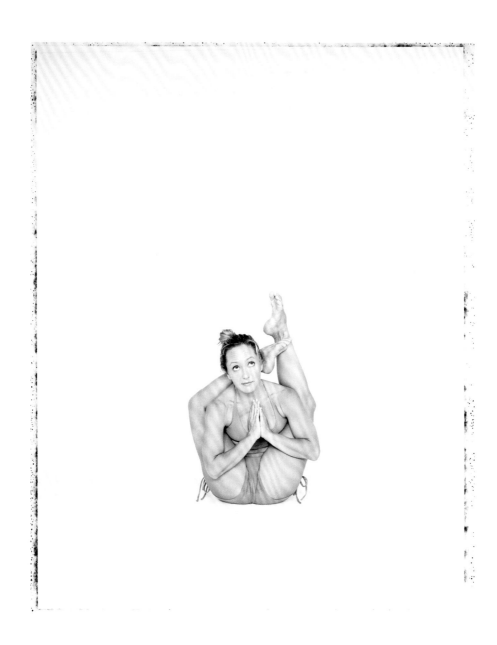

Bhuja Daṇḍāsana

भुजदण्डासन

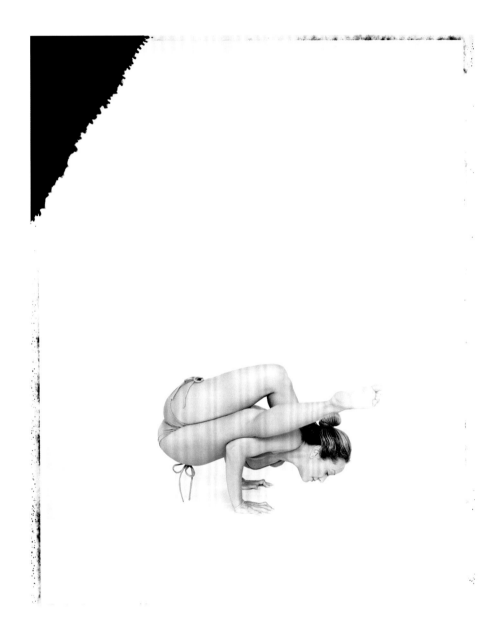

Pārśva Daṇḍāsana

पार्श्वदण्डासन

Adho Daṇḍāsana

ऊर्ध्वदण्डासन

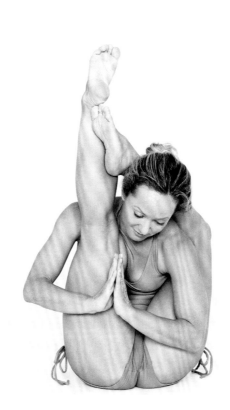

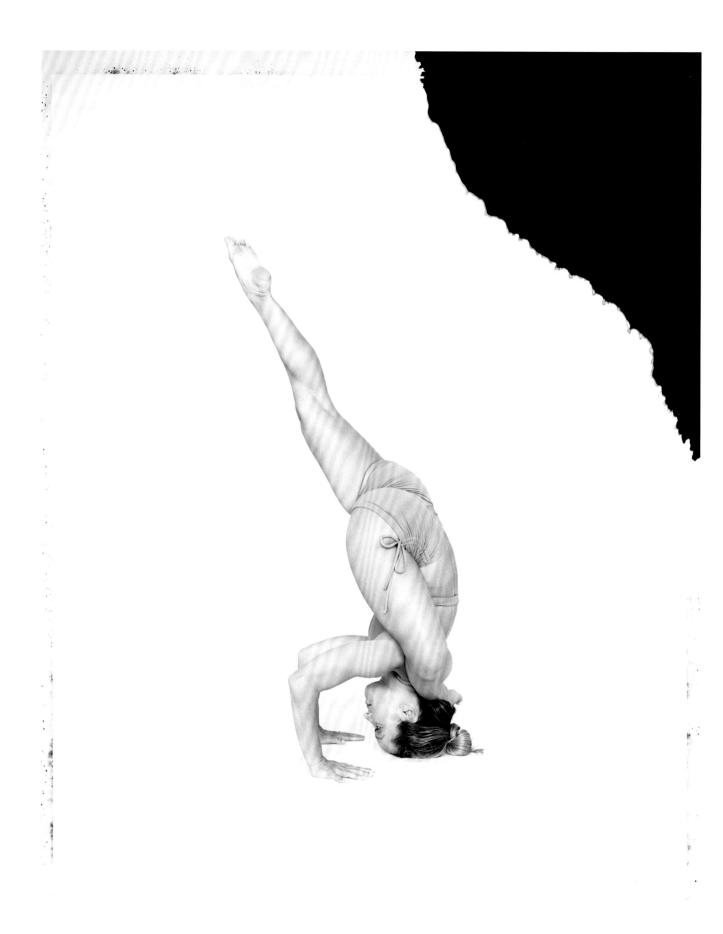

Ūrdhva Daṇḍasāna

ऊर्ध्वदण्डमान

Sama Koṇāsana

समकोणासन

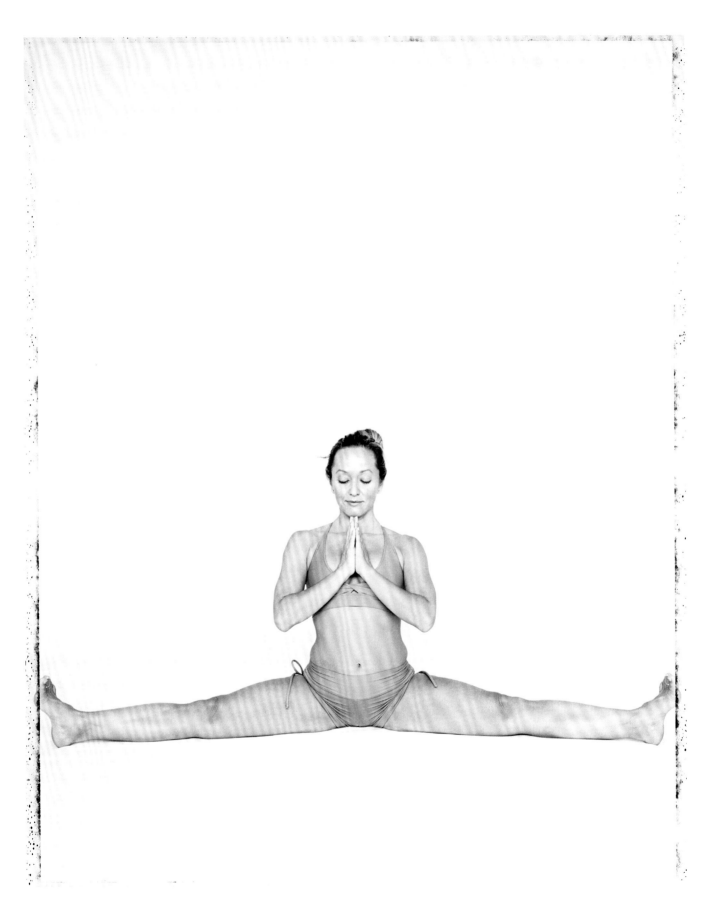

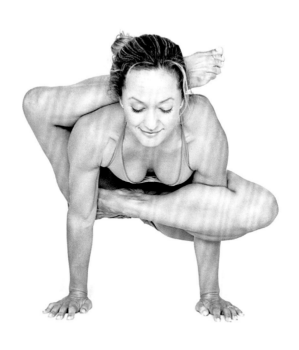

Omkarāsana

ओम्करासन

Ūrdhva Dhanurāsana

ऊर्ध्वधनुरासन

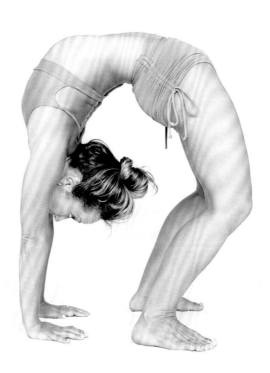

Finishing Sequence

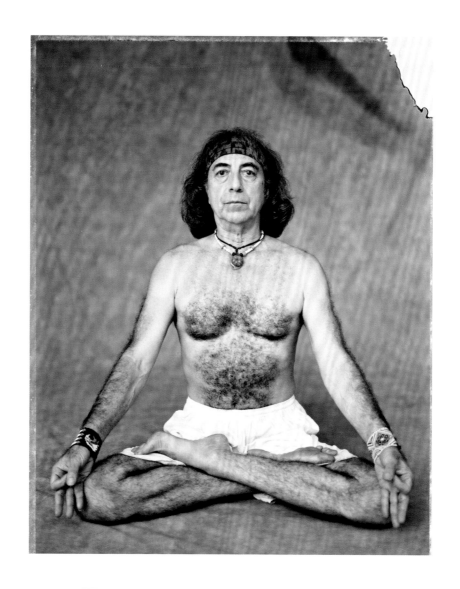

Danny Paradise

Love, The Path to be Taken

I'm not looking for the limelight
I follow my path
With clear goals in mind
With firm will in my backpack
It's love that moves me

Are you looking for the way?
Then join me for a while
When you open up,
Our paths will cross

The good heart is a force
Lively and inspiring
The clear eye is a compass
Focused and far-sighted

Every challenge is for growth
Determination needs intuition
To soften the character
Let me take you by the hand
I guide with love and responsibility

Sālamba Sarvāṅgāsana

सालम्बसर्वाङ्गासन

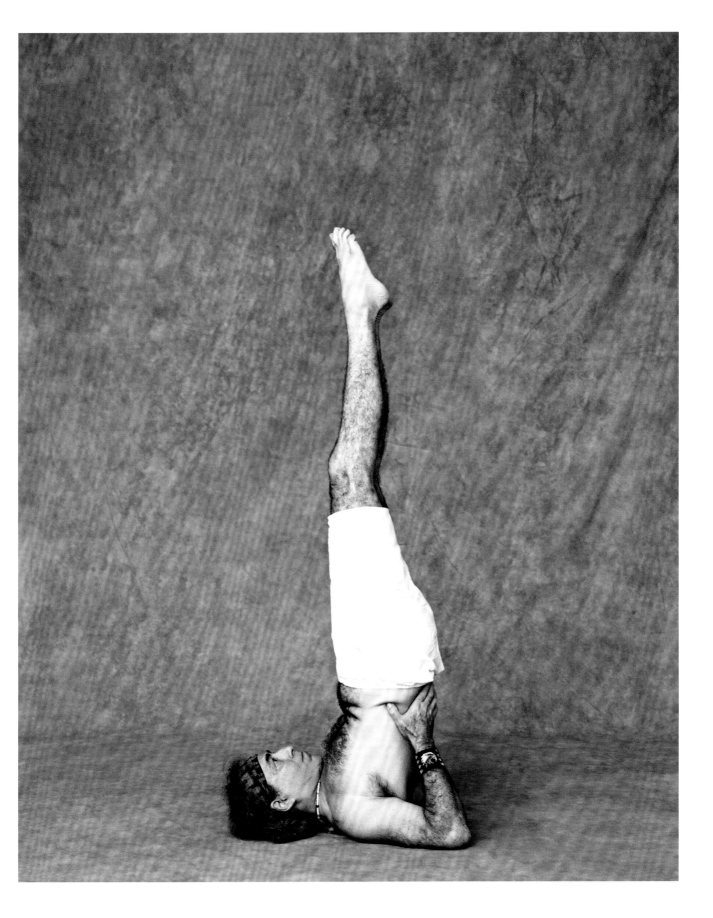

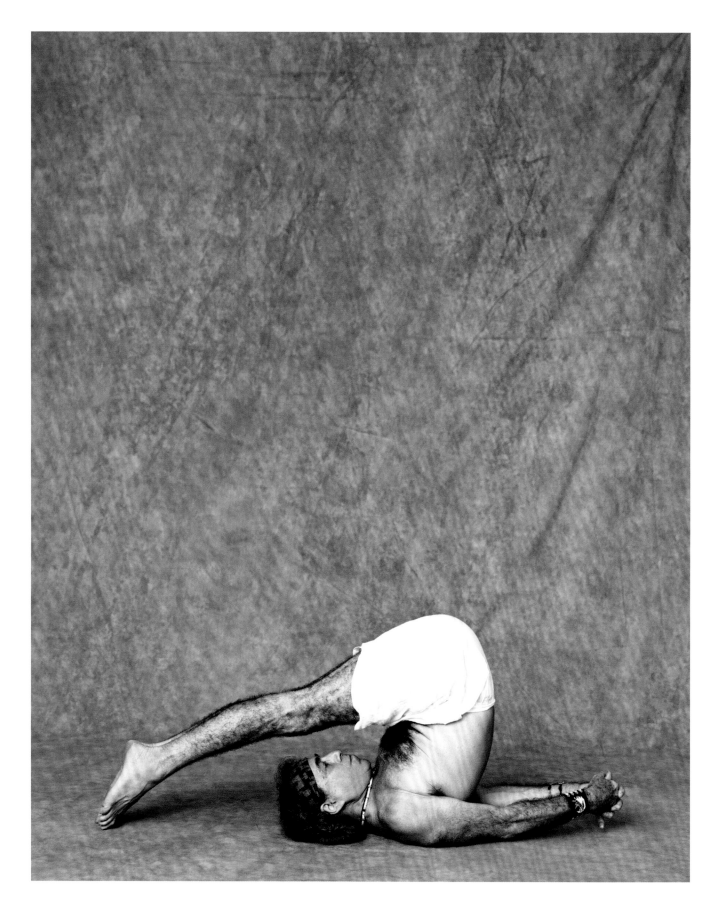

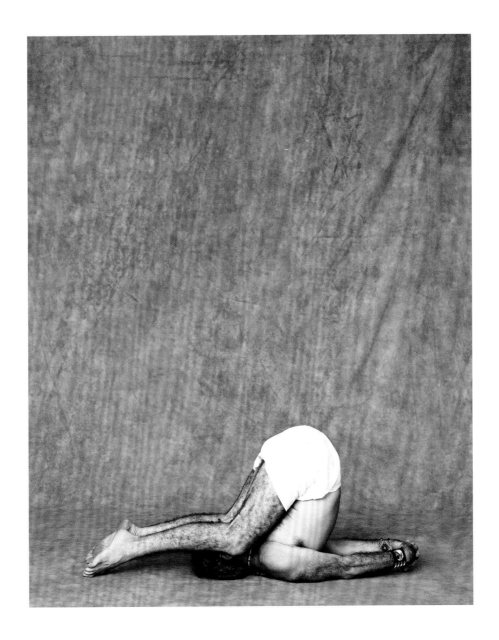

Karṇa Pīḍāsana

कर्णपीडासन

<

Halāsana

हलासन

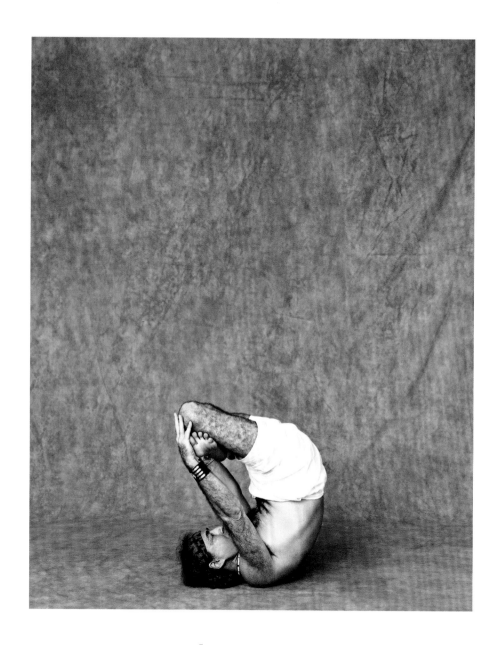

Ūrdhva Padmāsana

ऊर्ध्वपद्मासन

>

Piṇḍāsana

पिण्डासन

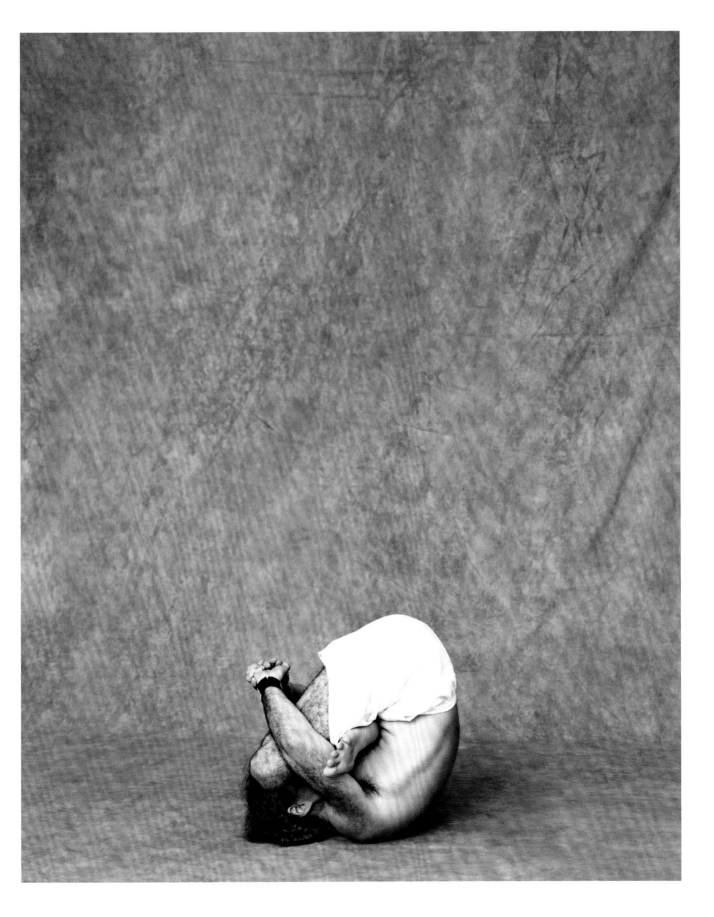

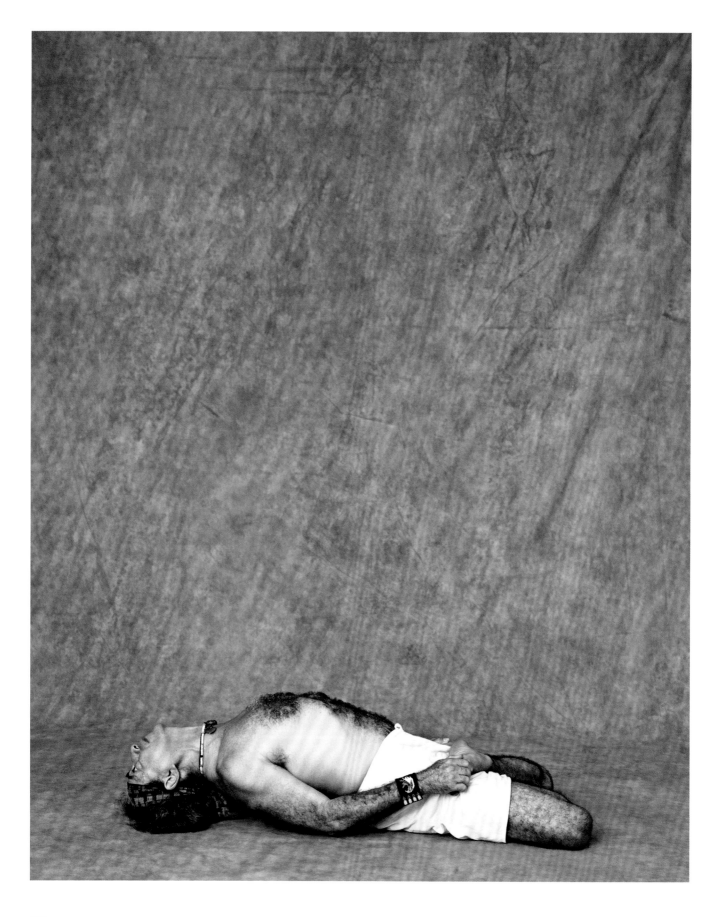

Matsyāsana

मत्स्यासन

Uttāna Pādāsana

उत्तानपादासन

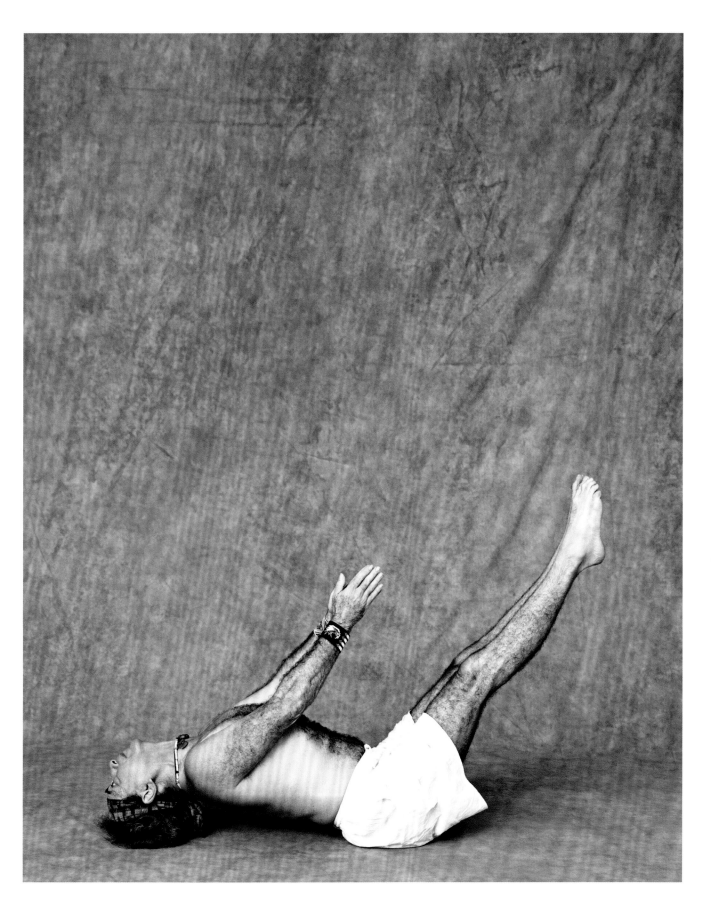

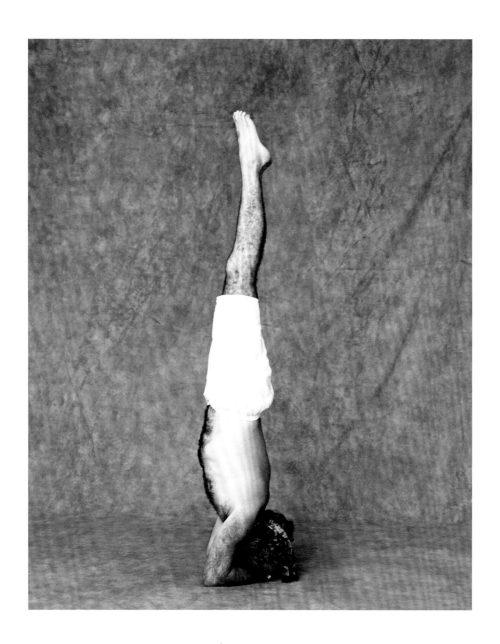

Śīrṣāsana A

कर्णपीडासन १

>

Ūrdhva Daṇḍāsana

ऊर्ध्वदण्डासन

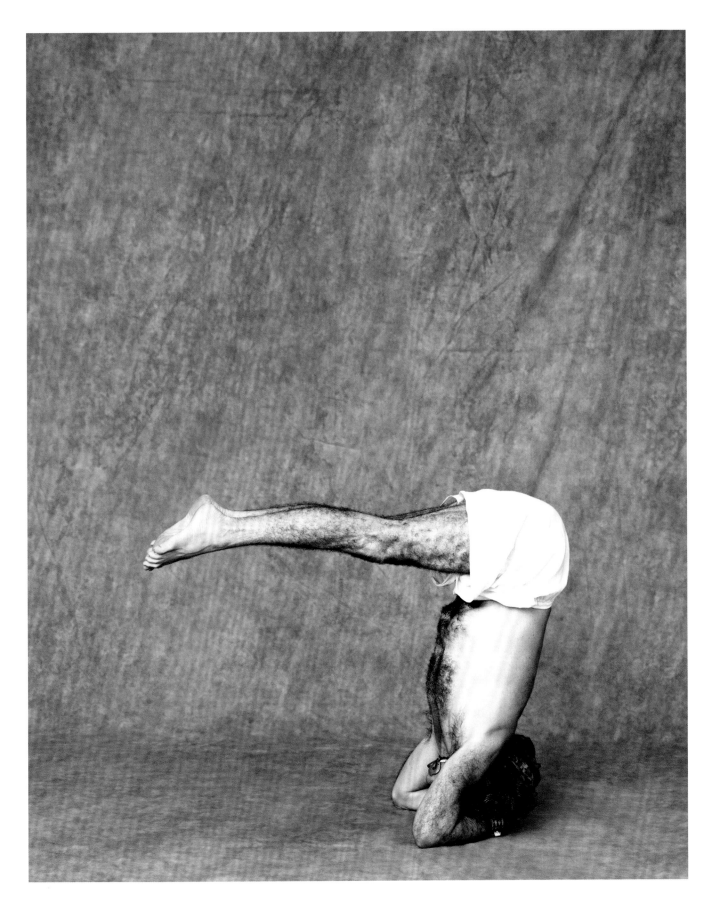

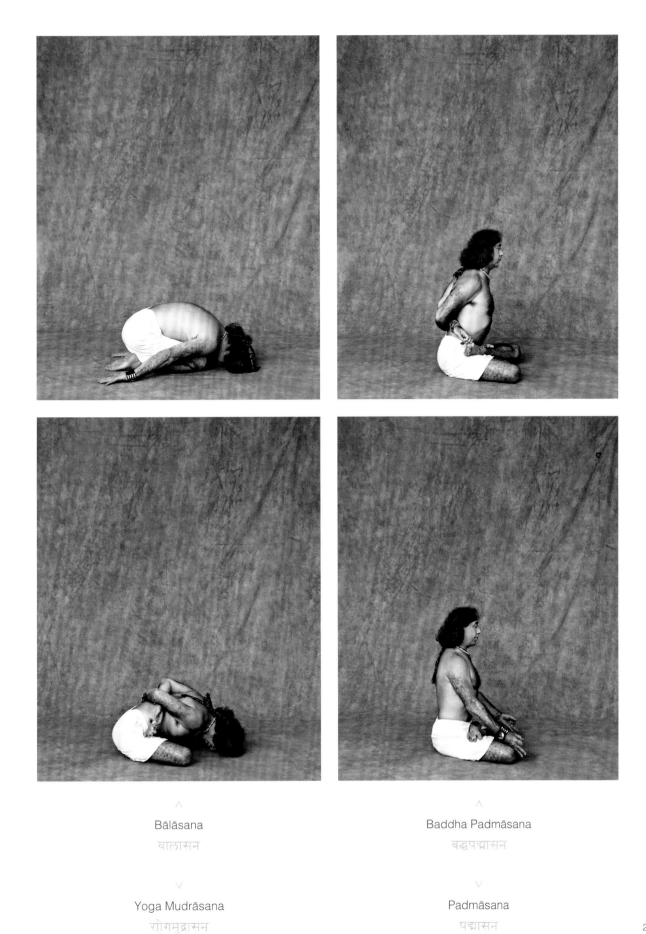

∧

Bālāsana

बालासन

∨

Yoga Mudrāsana

योगमुद्रासन

∧

Baddha Padmāsana

बद्धपद्मासन

∨

Padmāsana

पद्मासन

269

Utplutiḥ

उत्प्लुतिः

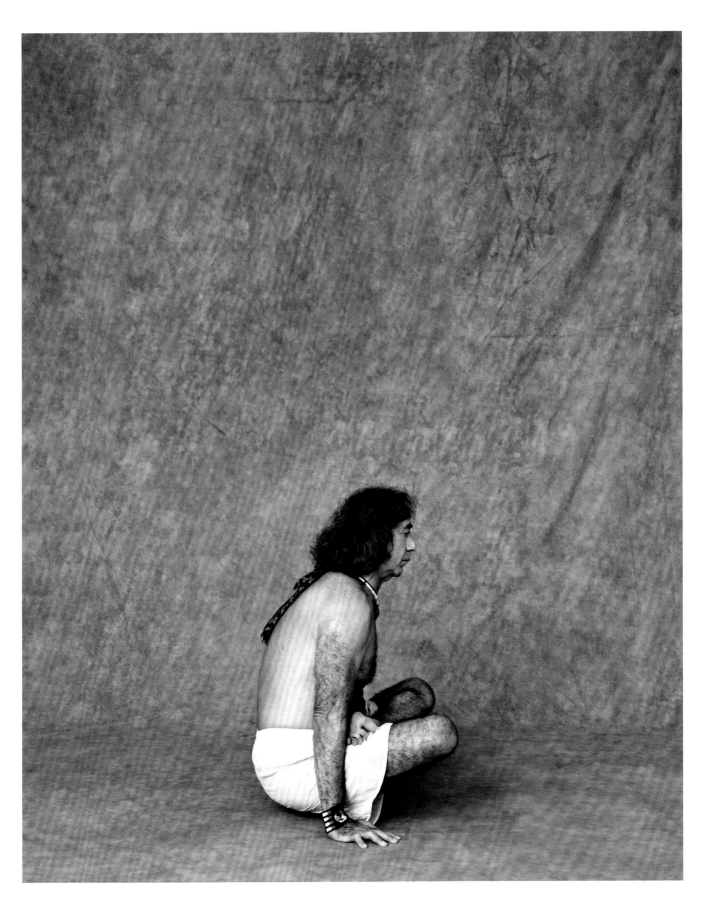

श्रीमद्भगवद्गीता

Shavasana

Śavāsana

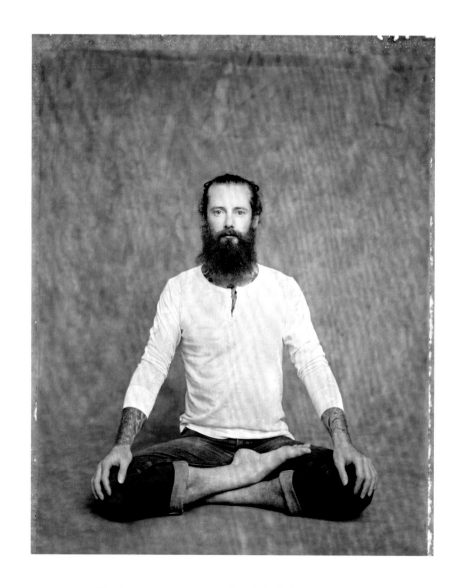

Richard Pilnick

Loneliness
Where closed eyes rest
Feet to take me away
Where no looks judge me

Insight
Where open eyes dance
Feet to take me to myself
My looks are filled with wonder

Follow your instinct
And you're a survivor
Flee from your expectations
And you're a refugee
Follow your talents
And you're a creator of the heart

Humanity
It's people who irritate me
Alienating myself from others
But it's love I want to give

Escapism
Adore the monks
But solitude can be a prison
Inventive ideas need to shine

Give eyes hands
The flair for captivating people
Broaden horizons
The authority over things unseen

Śavāsana

शासन

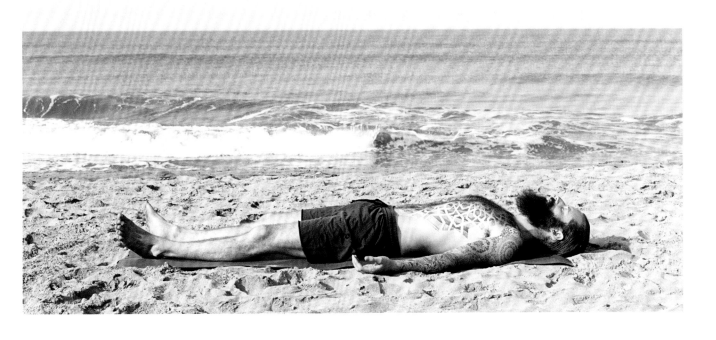

गुरु

The Teachers

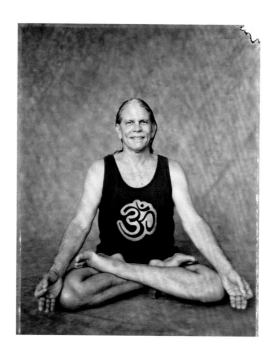

David Williams has been practising yoga daily, without interruption, since 1971, the last forty of them on the island of Maui, Hawaii. He is responsible for teaching the Ashtanga yoga system to many of today's leading teachers and practitioners, including Danny Paradise, David Swenson, Doug Swenson, Clifford Sweatte, Cliff Barber, Baptiste Marceau, Bryan Kest, Jonny Kest, Kathy Cooper, Andrew Eppler, Kathy McNames, Erica McHugh, and Ricky Tran.

In 1972, David met Manju Jois, the son of K. Pattabhi Jois, and saw him demonstrate the Ashtanga yoga primary series. This was at Dr. Swami Gitananda's Ananda Ashram in Pondicherry, South India, where David received his six-month yoga teachers training course certification. The following year, David began learning Ashtanga yoga from Pattabhi Jois at his home in Mysore, India. He was the first non-Indian to be taught the complete Ashtanga system of asanas and pranayama directly from him. In 1974, David became one of the first non-Indians to be certified to teach the Ashtanga yoga asanas and one of very few people certified by Jois to teach the pranayama.

www.ashtangayogi.com

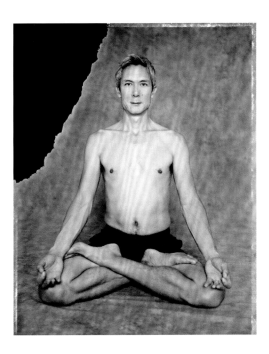

Gingi Lee has played a key role in popularizing Ashtanga yoga in the UK and has taught, trained and inspired many British yoga teachers. In 1997, he founded the Shala studio, one of London's first dedicated Ashtanga yoga centres, and he continues to teach there as one of Britain's most senior Ashtanga teachers.

Gingi studied and taught martial arts with his father, Sensei Richard Taibong, before he discovered yoga during a trip to India in 1989. In the Tar desert, Rajasthan, he was taught postures, pranayama and meditation under yoga master Swami Shyam, and saw that yoga was his true path. Discovering Ashtanga Vinyasa yoga, he was instantly drawn to the synchronicity of flowing breath to posture, and to the grace and strength of the practice. After completing a teacher-training course in Goa, he apprenticed for two years with Derek Ireland. He continued his studies with K. Pattabhi Jois in Mysore, before attending a two-year teacher training course with Graeme Northfield.

For 25 years, Gingi has focused his energy on teaching at the Shala, as well as hosting yoga workshops abroad. In 2017, he established the Shala School of Yoga teacher training programme with co-teachers Kath Roberts, Mark Kan and Norman Blair. A highly respected teacher, Gingi remains at the forefront of the yoga community. He regards Ashtanga as a living tradition, and is honoured to be among the teachers who have been instrumental in carrying it forward to the next generation of teachers and students.

www.theshalalondon.com

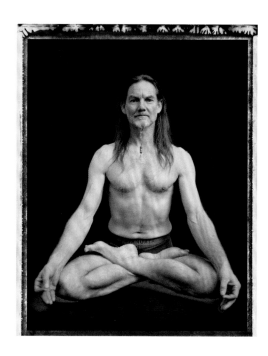

John Scott plays an influential role in growing the yoga community by travelling the world passing on the Vinyasa Counting Method of Ashtanga – learning to count in the language of his host while sharing the Sanskrit language of yoga.

John has been studying Ashtanga Vinyasa yoga since 1987, having been introduced to the practice by pioneering teachers Derek Ireland and Radha Warell in Skyros, Greece. This had a profound effect on him and he formed a close relationship with Derek, who guided him east to Mysore – where he began studies with K. Pattabhi Jois that continued until his teacher's passing in 2009. John maintains his close relationship with the family through Manju Jois, who he has known for many years.

His time spent with Pattabhi Jois has directly influenced John's teaching, and he remains greatly absorbed by the Vinyasa Counting Method he studied. He sees it as central to *tristana* (mind, body, breath synchonicity) and the capacity for the practice to become a moving meditation and a key to the eight-limb path. It is through the combination of Ashtanga Vinyasa yoga and deep enquiry into the self that John has brought all his experiences and meditations into his life work of sharing.

John wishes to acknowledge with great love and gratitude his first teacher, Derek Ireland, who guided him to India and connected him directly to the source of his practice.

www.johnscottyoga.com

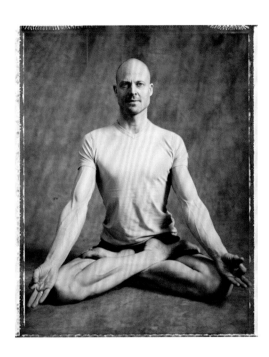

Dr. Ronald Steiner is the founder of AYI®. He is a sports physician, a researcher with focus on prevention of injury and rehabilitation, and one of the most well-known practitioners of Ashtanga yoga. He is also one of the few yoga teachers authorized in the traditional way by both Indian grand masters K. Pattabhi Jois and B.N.S. Iyengar.

As creator of the – possibly first – internet platform showing detailed photos of all four series from Ashtanga yoga, he played an influential role in spreading this practice throughout the world. Starting in 1998, countless practitioners have and still are using the freely provided "cheat sheets", checking the Vinyasa count or the proper Sanskrit name of an Asana. AYI has grown into one of the most comprehensive information resources for Ashtanga yoga. You can even join online yoga classes, learn Sanskrit or dive into the most important source texts of yoga there.

The AYI Method links traditional Ashtanga yoga with innovative yoga therapy and a modern view on yoga philosophy: in which the body and mind join together and find a harmonious balance. The practice is deeply rooted in the age-old tradition and keeps it alive. At the same time, AYI integrates the latest scientific findings in the fields of movement science, therapy, psychology, teaching methodology and Indological philosophy.

www.ashtangayoga.info / www.ayi.info

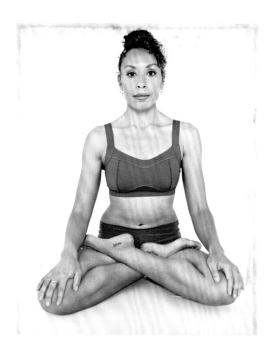

Laruga Glaser directs the Ashtanga yoga programme at Yogayama in Stockholm, Sweden, and teaches workshops and retreats internationally. An Advanced Level practitioner and student of yoga, as well as a Level 2 Teacher Certified with KPJAYI, Laruga entered into teaching after years of sustained practice and has been dedicated to Ashtanga yoga for more than 20 years.

Having been fascinated by mind/body connections from a young age, Laruga made her first connection with yoga and yoga philosophy in 1996. When she stumbled upon Ashtanga yoga she began her true journey, immersing herself in devoted studies. After ten years of established practice, she made the first of a dozen journeys to Mysore, India, to study at the K. Pattabhi Jois Ashtanga Yoga Institute. She studied under the guidance of K. Pattabhi Jois – who she considers her principal teacher and greatest influence – and his grandson R. Sharath Jois.

Laruga is dedicated to teaching the method of Ashtanga yoga to its fullest capacity, cultivating transparency in the tradition and continuing the deeply rich lineage of the practice, known as *parampara*. She teaches as an act of deep sharing and love for what yoga develops in each individual, facilitating the space to open, challenge and inspire students to realize their inherent potential.

www.larugayoga.com

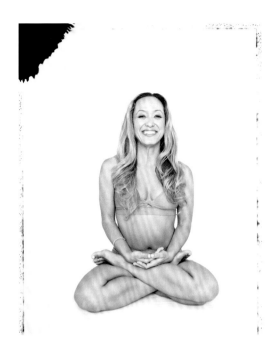

Kino MacGregor is an internationally acclaimed yoga teacher, inspirational speaker and author, who is the founder of Omstars – the world's first yoga TV network – and co-founder of the Miami Life Center. She now has more than 20 years of experience in Ashtanga and 18 years in Vipassana meditation.

Kino travelled to India as a 23-year-old, on the first of what would become annual pilgrimages. She is one of a select group of people to receive the certification to teach Ashtanga yoga from its founder K. Pattabhi Jois in Mysore, India, and to practise into the Fifth Series of Ashtanga yoga under R. Sharath Jois.

Ashtanga yoga is for Kino a way of life founded on a firm commitment to the moral and ethical precepts of truth, non-violence and love – being strong in yoga is not about a powerful handstand or a deep backbend, but is instead a daily ritual where people can tune in deeply to their spiritual centre. She believes that yoga should be accessible to everyone, and that the international community of yogis are responsible for maintaining the integrity of the sacred heart of yoga.

With more than one million followers on Instagram and more than 500,000 subscribers on YouTube and Facebook, Kino's message of spiritual strength is able to reach people all over the world.

www.kinoyoga.com

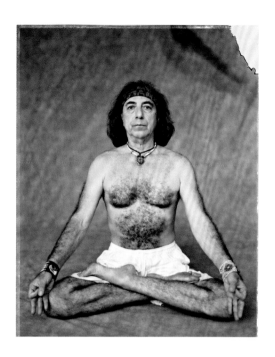

Danny Paradise has been practicing Ashtanga yoga since 1976 and has taught in 41 countries since 1979. He was the first Western 'travelling teacher' of Ashtanga yoga and has also introduced Ashtanga to some of the world's most renowned and talented musicians, actors, athletes, artists, designers, activists and film directors – including Sting, Trudie Styler, Madonna, Paul Simon, Edie Brickell, Marcel Marceau, Graham Nash, Eddie Vedder, Jeff Ament, Micky Hart, Bob Weir, Yusuf Islam (Cat Stevens), Donna Karan, Luciano Pavarotti, Lyle Lovett, Chris Botti, Dominic Miller, John McEnroe and Patty Smyth.

Danny initially studied with David Williams and Nancy Gilgoff – the first Western teachers and adepts of Ashtanga yoga from 1976 to 1981 learning Primary, Intermediate, Advanced A and B series. In 1978 and 1980, he was taught by K. Pattabhi Jois. As an advanced practitioner and teacher, Danny played a seminal role in communicating the Ashtanga form around the world through public classes. Danny also studied martial arts since he was 13 years old.

Danny recognizes yoga as an ancient Shamanic practice, with the basic premise that nature is our spiritual guide and teacher. He draws on diverse sources – the teachings of Krishnamurti, Buddha, Taoism and Ancient Egypt. Danny also shares the contemporary teachings of Carolyne Myss, Marianne Williamson, Shamanic indigenous cultures including Mayan, Hawaiian and Native American. His classes include non-dogmatic explorations of modifications, derivative routines and poses interspersed with Egyptian root yoga, kung fu and tai chi – all within the structure of the routines of Ashtanga yoga.

Danny understands yoga as ancestral suggestions – 'Soul Work' – designed to create freedom, evolution, well-being, and to help people fulfill their personal destiny, learn to age with peace, vitality, energy and grace. Danny is also a musician, songwriter, film maker and Human rights activist.

www.dannyparadise.com

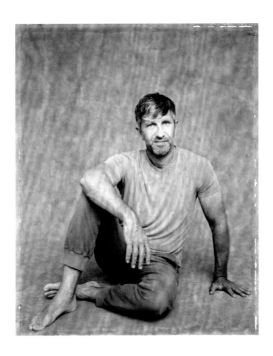

Eric Standop is a face reader, bestselling author and international keynote speaker. He is the founder of the Face Reading Academy, and has lectured in more than 20 countries to audiences in fields ranging from finance to health and wellness. He trained under three legendary masters to himself become a Master Face Reader who fluidly merges Chinese and South American face-reading methodologies; Greek techniques in physiognomy; and modern studies in micro-expressions and health and nutritional diagnosis.

Eric stumbled on the ancient art of face reading when trying to heal himself. After working in a high-pressure role in Germany as a PR and marketing director, he was forced to give up his job through stress and ill-health. He set off to travel the world in an attempt to restore his well-being, and met a face reader in South Africa who instantly diagnosed the source of his ailments. This set Eric on a new path. Seeking to develop his own face-reading skills, he travelled to Hong Kong to find a Chinese master willing to instruct him. He served a rigorous six-year apprenticeship before being inducted into the circle of *sifus*, accomplished Chinese master readers.

Eric's astute diagnostic abilities have made him the go-to advisor for many powerful decision-makers, as well as individuals who seek to understand themselves better. Through teaching people to see themselves as clearly as he does, Eric helps his clients to deeper self-understanding and acceptance, and gives them the confidence to begin making positive changes in their lives.

www.ericstandop.com

Acknowledgments

The author would like to thank, in no particular order:

Ganesha: for introducing me to yoga in Gokarna, India, in 2009; Shiva Shankar: the first yogi I photographed in Gokarna, India, in 2012; Cat & Phil Douglas (www.sangyeyoga.com): for their portrait that was hung in the National Portrait Gallery in London in 2013 and 2014, and which cemented my yoga photography journey; Marco Aicardi (www.ashtangagokarna.weebly.com): for introducing me to Ashtanga yoga in Gokarna, India, in 2014.

Cornelia Sailer, Munich, Germany, and Clare Lim, co-director of SharedSpace (www.sharedspace.hk), Hong Kong: for their support in helping to fund this project from the beginning; Richard Chan and Chan Photographic Imaging (www.chanphotographicimaging.co.uk): for their support and generosity in developing the film for this project; Dr. Ronald Steiner (www.ashtangayoga.info): for providing the Sanskrit text and asana names; Barb Wilson (www.bwfineprint.co.uk): my master printer.

Selina and Ulrich: for providing me with the space to photograph Laruga Glaser; Francesca Maniglio and Yoga in Salento (www.yogainsalento.com): for giving me the space to shoot Danny Paradise and David Williams in your beautiful retreat. Benji from Sacred Heart Centre, Edinburgh (www.sacredheartcentre.org). Miami Life Centre for the space to photograph Kino MacGregor.

And, of course, to David Williams, Gingi Lee, John Scott, Dr. Ronald Steiner, Laruga Glaser, Kino MacGregor, Danny Paradise, Eric Standop and Matthew Clark.

First published 2019 by
Ammonite Press
an imprint of Guild of Master Craftsman Publications Ltd
Castle Place, 166 High Street, Lewes, East Sussex, BN7 1XU, United Kingdom

Text and Photographs © Richard Pilnick, 2019
Poems © Eric Standop, 2019
Sanskrit © Dr. Ronald Steiner, 2019
Introduction © Matthew Clark, 2019
Copyright in the Work © GMC Publications Ltd, 2019

ISBN 978 1 78145 367 4

The publishers and author can accept no legal responsibility for any consequences arising from the application of information, advice or instructions given in this publication. NOTE: Not all exercises are suitable for everyone. Consult your professional healthcare provider before beginning a new exercise programme.

A catalogue record for this book is available from the British Library.

Publisher: Jason Hook
Design Manager: Robin Shields
Editor: Jamie Pumfrey

Colour reproduction by GMC Reprographics
Printed and bound in China

AMMONITE
PRESS

www.ammonitepress.com

How was the book? Please post you feedback and photos: #ashtangayoga